THE ORIGIN OF CANCER

and

Its Causes & Prevention

By

Phil Matsumoto

Originofcancer.com

DEDICATION

This book is dedicated to my father, Tsuyoshi Matsumoto, who loved his family and who loved books, and was an author himself, and to my mother, Emi Matsumoto, who was an "education mom," who really pushed me to get a great education and sacrificed much to do so. This book is also dedicated to my sister, brother-in-law, nephew and his wife, and the rest of my family, without whose support, I wouldn't have been able to finish this book, and all the friends, colleagues, teachers, etc., who made a huge contribution to the completion of this work.

TABLE OF CONTENTS

A Synopsis of our Theory on the Origin of Cancer

We believe that you have to return to when life first originated on Earth about 4 billion years ago to discover how cancer originated. When you do that, you discover many fascinating connections between cancer and the origin of life. An important clue that prompted us to begin this journey was how cancer cells resemble bacteria in many ways (for example, see the section on HeLa cells on page 84), and bacteria and viruses were the first lifeforms to evolve. This is why we began to focus our attention on bacteria and viruses.

The mycoplasma bacteria forms an important part of our theory on the origin of cancer. We were very fortunate to find an article on mycoplasma on Wikipedia (please do a search on Wikipedia for mycoplasma), which explains how the mycoplasma bacteria are responsible for many different kinds of cancer, such as breast cancer, colon cancer, stomach cancer, renal (kidney) cancer, and prostate cancer. We were also fortunate to find an article on cholesterol that points out how the mycoplasma bacteria are one of the few bacteria that uses cholesterol. (Cholesterol is a factor, not only in heart disease, but also in cancer. See this article on cholesterol and cancer from the University of Alberta: https://medicalxpress.com/news/2016-04-bad-cholesterol-production-growth-tumours.html)

Another important clue was a picture of a methanogenic bacteria (see page 91) that we found that shows their internal sterol membranes. These archaebacteria were the inventors of sterol membranes, which eventually became incorporated into the outer membranes of many eukaryotic cells that evolved after this, including human cells.

According to biologist Lynn Margulis, mycoplasma was the host bacterium for the endosymbiotic merging of the bacteria that formed the first eukaryotic cells, or cells that have a separate and distinct nucleus. (See the graphic below from biologist Lynn Margulis of the mycoplasma merging with the bdellovibrio [which is called "Aerobic bacteria" in the illustration below], which became the mitochondria, to form the first eukaryotic cell. This agrees perfectly with our theory.) This means that every eukaryotic cell that evolved after this was a descendant of these cancer-causing bacteria, and this is why cancer occurs in many different organisms, and not just in humans.

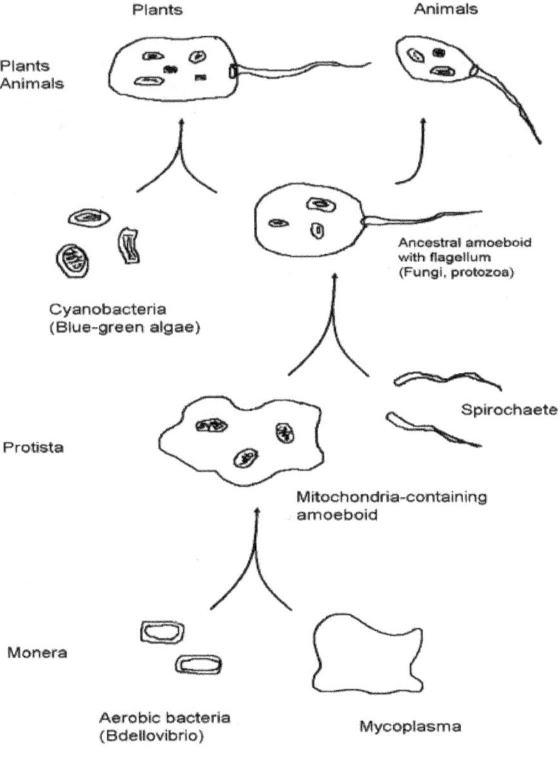

Source: Lynn Margulis

Other relevant Wikipedia articles (please search on Wikipedia using these terms):

Archaebacteria

Infectious Causes of Cancer

Methanogens (Methane producers)

Methanosarcina (Methane producers)

Methylotrophs (Methane eaters)

Nitrosamines

THE ORIGIN OF CANCER
AND ITS CAUSES & PREVENTION

INTRODUCTION

For the first time ever, there is a plausible theory on the origin of cancer. We will take you back through the dark mists of time to solve one of the greatest mysteries of the ages: Where does cancer come from and why does it exist? We will give you a timeline on the origin of life on this planet and show you where the origin of cancer lies along that timeline. By understanding how cancer originated, we will be able to explain why certain factors cause cancer and why other factors prevent cancer (and why it seems like just about everything causes cancer). This new theory is simple, elegant, and comprehensive because it provides an explanation for why certain things cause cancer and not just how they cause cancer. There have been many new discoveries in the past few decades in the fields of cancer research, the origin of life, microbiology, and DNA research, but no one has brought all of these new facts together into a credible theory on the origin of cancer—until now.

We hope that this new understanding of cancer will accelerate the development of new ways to prevent and treat cancer and will help reduce the number of people in this country who will be diagnosed with cancer every year, which is now about 1.8 million,1 and the number of lives claimed by this disease, which is currently about 600,000.

Cancer is the second leading cause of death in the United States after heart disease. It is estimated that men have a one-in-two lifetime risk of developing cancer and women have a one-in-three risk. The current scientific evidence indicates that about one-third of all cancers are related to nutrition and other lifestyle factors and are therefore preventable; only an estimated 5 to 10% of cancers are considered to be hereditary. Fortunately, more than half of all people diagnosed with cancer will be cured.

Cancer research is continuously progressing which makes it difficult to present information that won't soon become obsolete. As more becomes known about cancer, researchers realize how little they really know about it. We don't claim to have all the answers–cancer is a complex and multi-factorial subject; in fact, it is actually more than 200 diseases.

We will close this book with an extensive bibliography for our readers who want to learn more about cancer and review the actual sources for our revolutionary new theory on the origin of cancer.

CHAPTER 1

WHAT IS CANCER?

Cancer is a malignant or uncontrolled growth of undifferentiated cells in the body. In many respects, cancer cells resemble the most primitive life forms on Earth. They can sometimes exhibit amoeba-like movement. They can create the energy they need to live by glycolysis, which is a more primitive way of deriving energy from sugar that doesn't require oxygen. In fact, cancer cells can exist for days in a cyanide atmosphere totally devoid of oxygen, which may be what our atmosphere was like billions of years ago when life first formed on Earth. Later, we will explain what these characteristics mean and why cancer cells exhibit them.

CANCER CELLS ARE IMMORTAL

As long as they receive nutrients, cancer cells can live and multiply without end.

A tumor removed from a woman who died over six decades ago is still living in the laboratory and providing cancer cells for experimentation. (See the "Hela" cells section in Chapter Six for more information on these cancer cells.)

CANCER CELLS LACK "CONTACT INHIBITION"

Cancer cells don't stop growing when one layer of cells touches another layer, like normal cells do. Some cancer cells resemble fetal and neonatal cells in that they divide quickly, and you don't know what kind of cell they are going to be until they begin to differentiate into the specialized cells that make up the arms, the legs, the eyes, the gastrointestinal tract, and so on. Cancer cells, however, do not differentiate. They look unlike normal cells when examined under a microscope. Many cancer cells resemble amorphous masses with claws or tentacles, which is why this disease is named after the crab.

Contrary to popular belief, most cancer cells do not grow faster than normal cells (fetal cells being normal cells). Instead, the reason they appear to do so is because they reproduce at the same rate or slightly slower than normal cells, but they don't die off like normal cells. Cancer cells can die; in fact, most tumors contain necrotic[2] tissue in their centers as the tumors outgrow the nutrients supplied to them. Cancer cells need fewer nutrients than normal cells to live, but a tumor can sometimes quickly outgrow the network of newly-created blood vessels that supply it. The size of a tumor in the body can double in as little as four days or in as many as 500 days. (The blood cancers—leukemia and lymphoma, or cancer of the lymph glands—reproduce at the fastest rates.) A tumor can actually contain quite a large proportion of normal cells, or it can consist mostly of dead tissue in its center surrounded by living and reproducing cancer cells on the outside.

CELLS IN OUR BODY ARE TURNING CANCEROUS EVERY DAY

Normal cells are continually transforming into cancer cells in our bodies all the time3, but our immune system, if it is working properly, is able to destroy these cancer cells before they can divide and grow into palpable tumors. The mechanism by which the immune system destroys cancer cells is fascinating. From the book, *Nutrition, Health, and Disease*, by Gary Price Todd, M.D. (1985 The Donning Co.), we learn how the body destroys cancer cells:

"…The living lymphocyte… is an astounding cell. In a culture containing cancer cells, the lymphocyte could be seen entering each cell, going directly to the nucleus of the cell and apparently inspecting it. If the cell were a normal cell, the lymphocyte left just as it entered; through the cell wall.

"Amazingly, the cell wall which had just opened to allow the lymphocyte into the interior of the cell closed without a trace of the opening. If the cell were cancerous, however, an even more astounding thing happened: The normally spherical lymphocyte pulled back from the nucleus of the cancerous cell, assumed the shape of a torpedo, and plunged deep into the depths of the offending cell's nucleus, immediately exploding and disintegrating both the lymphocyte and the cancerous cell! It was something out of Star Wars. You would have to see it to believe it. The phase photography movie clearly demonstrated this many times.

"Very obviously, our bodies have sophisticated mechanisms for destroying cancerous cells, just as we have systems designed to destroy bacteria and viruses. With such a mechanism in daily operation, there must be a need. I believe that we daily produce cancerous cells in the normal routine of repair and reproduction of cells, and the lymphocytes serve to eliminate those cells before they multiply and destroy us.

"That being the case, it would appear that cancer is the result not so much of carcinogenic substances producing cancerous cells, as the failure of normal immune mechanisms to eliminate those cells. True, substances which increase the likelihood of mutation of a dividing cell may serve to overwhelm the immune system, but after a few prudent efforts to eliminate the obvious offenders, we should spend our efforts in looking for ways to enhance our natural immune systems, rather than trying to eliminate from our environment every suspect chemical. If we search hard enough, we will find that the world is full of natural carcinogens…"

As we will see in the next chapter, there are literally thousands of carcinogens.

CANCER CELLS CAN ACT LIKE AMOEBAE

Cancer cells can exhibit amoeboid motion, which means that they can squeeze through blood vessel walls like an amoeba and move to other parts of the body in a process called metastasis.

CANCER CELLS ARE HIGHER IN SODIUM THAN NORMAL CELLS

Our bodies try to maintain a continuous balance between certain elements at all times. One important set of these elements is sodium and potassium. Potassium is important for proper muscle functioning, and is especially critical for the heart muscles. Cancer cells are higher in sodium than normal cells. Vegetables and fruits are high in potassium in their fresh, unprocessed state. (Canned and frozen vegetables are usually much higher in salt than potassium, because salt is added by food processors.)

CANCER CELLS CAN HAVE MULTIPLE DNA

Some cancer cells have multiple nuclei. These cancer cells have too many strands of DNA in their nuclei.

CANCER CELLS GENERATE STEM CELLS AND FETAL PROTEINS

Some cancer cells produce stem cells, which are undifferentiated cells that have the potential to become any type of cell, such as a lung cell, a liver cell, a skin cell, and so on. Other cancer cells generate fetal proteins, which are proteins normally only seen as a fetus develops in the womb (or in vitro4).

CANCER CELLS EXHIBIT DRUG RESISTANCE

Cancer cells can develop a tolerance for the drugs that are used to treat them. It then becomes necessary to use a different drug to fight them, or a different combination of drugs. Some bacteria show this same characteristic; they can become tolerant to certain antibiotics and drugs used to control them.

CANCER CELLS CAN EXIST IN LOW OXYGEN ENVIRONMENTS

This characteristic was one of the first clues to us that it might prove beneficial to investigate the origin of life forms during the formative stages of this planet when very little oxygen existed in the atmosphere. In later chapters, we will explain which life forms we mean and how they might have given rise to cancer.

SUMMARY

Cancer cells are immortal. As long as they are given nutrients and the other necessities of life, they can live forever.

Cancer cells lack contact inhibition. They don't stop growing when they touch another cell or the edge of a petri dish.

Cancer cells can act like amoebae. They can move through their environment like single-celled creatures. Some cancer cells have multiple DNA.

Cancer cells can produce stem cells and fetal proteins.

Cancer cells can become resistant to antibiotics and other drugs.

Cancer cells can exist in a low-oxygen environment.

Cells are turning cancerous in our bodies every day, but our immune systems, if they are working correctly, can destroy them before they turn into large tumors that can spread.

CHAPTER 2

THE CAUSES OF CANCER

What causes cancer? Sometimes it seems like just about everything causes cancer–everything from overeating, or an excess of calories, fat, sugar, and protein, which appears to be responsible for such cancers as breast cancer and prostate cancer, to pollution, by poisons ranging from gasoline to vinyl chloride, which appears to be responsible for such cancers as liver and brain cancer. The list of cancer-causing chemicals is a mile long; in fact, in the book, *Cancer Causing Chemicals* (1981 Van Nostrand Reinhold), it fills 200 pages.

Edith Efron in her book, The Apocalyptics (1984 Simon & Schuster) sums up the situation eloquently:

"Industrial carcinogens are susceptible to political action; one can ban products, one can close factories. Hypothetically, the whole Industrial Revolution could be turned off. But the carcinogens that have been reported here cannot be turned off; if the data or any significant portion of them are valid, they are expressions of laws of nature and even Congress in its wisdom cannot repeal them. This carcinogenic hell, the scientists are telling us, is the planet earth itself, and we cannot escape it. It is, consequently, a more awesome picture.

"It is also a picture of mind-boggling complexity. We see that carcinogens are reported to be every kind of thing: They are motionless crystals, flowing gases, liquids. They are everywhere: They rain down upon us from the skies, they radiate upward from crevices beneath the sea, from the rocks and the soil, they flow through the veins of plants and trees, they gush out in torrents from forests.

They are alive: They grow, they crawl, they bloom, they blossom. And they are inside us: They are part of our vital physiological processes; they course through our bloodstream, they are in our saliva, in our digestive tracts. We inhale them, we drink them, and we feed on them ceaselessly, and in the act of absorbing them, we renew the needed supply in our bodies, for we cannot live without them; we ourselves are carcinogenic and radioactive beings. And even the act of dying is carcinogenic, for putrefaction, whether of plant or of animal, breeds new carcinogens. Were we to perish on a fiery bier, our broiling tissues and the very ash to which we were reduced would be carcinogenic. If these extraordinary data are valid, they tell us that in some ungraspable way the entire universe is implicated in the disease that is known as cancer…"

IS CANCER REVERSIBLE OR CURABLE?

Yes, nature always seems to provide a way out; we just need to make the effort to look for it. The answer to this question can be found all around us and inside us and should soon become obvious to anybody who takes the time to observe and think: nature is the answer; nature can provide the cure. (We will explain what this means later.) As an example of how "easy" it is to reverse some cancers, leukemia cells can be fairly easily converted back into normal cells. As the article below, Cell Differentiation and Malignancy, explains, all it takes to cure leukemia is for the body to produce the right proteins–specifically, the

Macrophage and Granulocyte Inducer Proteins, MGI-1 and MGI-2.

Cell Differentiation and Malignancy

By Leo Sachs

Department of Genetics, Weizmann Institute of Science, Rehovot 76100, Israel

Abstract

"An understanding of the mechanism that controls growth and differentiation in normal cells would seem to be an essential requirement to elucidate the origin and reversibility of malignancy. For this approach I have mainly used normal and leukemic blood cells, and in most studies have used myeloid blood cells as a model system. Our development of systems for the in vitro cloning and clonal differentiation of normal blood cells made it possible to study the controls that regulate growth (multiplication) and differentiation of these normal cells and the changes in these controls in leukemia. Experiments with normal blood cell precursors have shown that normal cells require different proteins to induce growth and differentiation. We have also shown that in normal myeloid precursors, growth-inducing protein induces both growth and production of differentiation-inducing protein so this ensures the coupling between growth and differentiation that occurs in normal development. The origin of malignancy involves uncoupling of growth and differentiation. This can be produced by changes from inducible to constitutive expression of specific genes that result in asynchrony in the coordination required for the normal developmental program. Normal myeloid precursors require an external source of growth-inducing protein for growth, and we have identified different types of leukemic cells. Some no longer require and others constitutively produce their own growth- inducing protein. But addition of the normal differentiation- inducing protein to these malignant cells still induces their normal differentiation, and the mature cells are then no longer malignant…"

THE CAUSES OF CANCER

CHEMICALS

There are literally thousands of different chemicals that cause cancer, and before now, no one has discovered a common thread that ties all of them together. We believe that we have found that common thread, and we'll tell you what it is in Chapters Six and Seven.

Here, briefly, is a list of some common chemicals that cause cancer:

Ammonia

Ammonia is believed to increase the risk of cancer, as the following excerpt from *Nutritional Factors in the Induction & Maintenance of Malignancy* by Denis Burkitt QZ200 N979 1982 (UCSD Biomedical Library) indicates:

"The form of cancer that has been most specifically linked with Western diets is that involving the large bowel. All available evidence points to excessive fat in the diet as a causative factor (Wynder and Reddy, 1975) and adequate fiber as protective (Cummings, 1982; Burkitt, 1971b; Walker and Burkitt, 1976).

Until recently, the former hypothesis was considered much the stronger, but during the last few years, the latter has been gaining increased acceptability.
"The mechanisms whereby dietary fiber is believed to protect against bowel cancer can be summarized as follows:

Dilution. Fiber, and cereal fiber in particular, increases fecal bulk and thus dilutes any fecal carcinogens.

Reducing contact time. By hastening passage of bowel contents, particularly through the colon, fiber reduces contact time between fecal carcinogens and the bowel mucosa.

Altering pH. By reducing fecal pH, fiber probably reduces bacterial degradation of cholesterol and primary bile acids into potential carcinogens. This has certainly been demonstrated in in vitro experiments (MacDonald et al., 1978).

Action of butyrate. Fiber increases butyrate, which has been shown to protect cells from malignant transformation (Hagopian et al., 1977).

Availability of ammonia. The proliferation of bacteria resulting from increased fiber intake uses up free nitrogen and thus reduces that available for ammonia formation. Ammonia is believed to increase susceptibility of cells to malignant transformation, so its reduction can be considered to be beneficial (Visek, 1972)."

The article above discusses how higher levels of bacteria are found in the colon with higher intakes of fiber, which result in lower levels of ammonia. Since ammonia is thought to increase the risk of cells turning cancerous, this would explain why populations that eat high fiber diets seem to have lower rates of colon cancer5.

Carbon Monoxide

Carbon monoxide is a strong tumor-creating gas, as the article below indicates. The reason why it causes brain tumors is because it is one of the few chemicals that can cross the "blood-brain barrier" that protects the brain from most toxic chemicals.

From *"Poison is My Profession"* by Gene Stone, Los Angeles Times Magazine, August 6, 1989:

"A family of Vietnamese refugees put charcoal in their fireplace and contracted carbon-monoxide poisoning; Bayer recommended that some of them be treated in hyperbaric chambers pumped with high levels of pure oxygen. The more pressing problem, the long- term effects of carbon-monoxide poisoning, was untreatable and could surface only a few weeks later in the form of a brain tumor."

Hydrochloric acid

Hydrochloric acid is carcinogenic, as the article below from *The Riddle of Cancer* by Charles Oberling 1952 Yale University Press QZ200 O123R (UCSD BML) indicates, although the experiment has been complicated by the addition of phthalic acid or 1, 2- benzene dicarboxylic acid. (A sarcoma is a cancer of connective tissue.)

"Very curious results were reported by Suntzeff, Babcock, and Leo Loeb. These investigators injected mice repeatedly with a dilute solution of hydrochloric acid adjusted to pH 5 by means of acid potassium phthalate. Of 8 mice thus treated 4 had sarcomas 10 to 16 months later at the site of the injections."

Hydrochloric acid and the other chemicals mentioned in this chapter seem to be random causes of cancer, but, in reality, all of these causative factors fit in with our theory on the origin of cancer. We'll tell you how they do so in Chapter Seven.

Nickel

Nickel dust breathed into the nasal passages and lungs causes cancer. Nickel is used in the manufacture of alkali batteries, ceramics, coins, and other products. It is also used as a catalyst in the hydrogenation process for fats and oils. In order to keep fats like soybean and cottonseed oil from turning rancid through oxidation (combining with oxygen), hydrogen gas is bubbled through these heated oils to bond with the sites on the oil molecules that would normally be filled by oxygen atoms. This creates a product that has a much longer shelf life and is more solid (like margarine). The most important fact to remember about nickel is that it is a "reducing" agent. (The significance of this will be explained in more detail in later chapters.)

Nitrosamines

Nitrosamines are found in foods such as bacon, beer, and in tobacco products.

They are formed when chemicals like sodium nitrite are added to foods to prevent botulism, which is a deadly form of food poisoning. These nitrites are converted into nitrosamines when they react with amines, which are organic derivatives of ammonia. Many types of nitrosamines exist and about 90% of them have been found to be carcinogenic in a wide variety of animals in the lab. The carcinogenic activity of nitrosamines can be prevented by the addition of vitamin C.

DIETARY CAUSES

Meats

In a study by the American Institute for Cancer Research, it was found that when meat is cooked, compounds called heterocyclic amines (HCAs) are formed that have been linked with increased cancer risk in some animal studies. Studies in the Journal of the National Cancer Institute have shown that people who eat lots of charred or well-done meat are three to five times more likely to develop breast, colon and stomach cancer than those who consume it less often. Studies on mice have demonstrated that these HCAs collect in breast tissue and can cause changes in DNA.

Rancid Fats

Over forty percent of the calories of the typical American diet are due to fat. Fats and cholesterol are oxidized during cooking. Rancid and oxidized fats contain a wide variety of carcinogens and promoters of cancer, such as fatty acid hydroperoxides, endoperoxides, cholesterol, and free radicals. The colon and digestive tract are continually being exposed to these fat-derived carcinogens. Human breast fluid can also contain high levels of cholesterol epoxide, which is an oxidized form of cholesterol. Some dietary fatty acids are also converted to hydrogen peroxide, which is a carcinogen and promoter of cancer, when these fatty acids are oxidized.

Americans consume about twelve grams of trans fatty acids and an equal amount of unnatural cis fatty acids, mainly from hydrogenated vegetable fats every day. There is some controversy about whether trans and cis fatty acids cause cancer; more research on these fats is being done.

FREE RADICALS

Free radicals are extremely reactive molecules with unpaired electrons. (Stable molecules have paired electrons.) They can damage DNA and cause wrinkling, premature aging, heart disease, cancer, and other diseases. Antioxidants like vitamin C and vitamin E prevent free radicals from exerting their damaging effects. (See the section on vitamins in Chapter Three for more information on how vitamins prevent free radicals.)

GENETICS

There is a genetic component to cancer as well, although it is probably not as large as most people think. Scientists estimate that about 5-10% of cancers have genetic causes. A good example of a cancer with a genetic cause is retinoblastoma, which is a form of eye cancer that children usually under the age of five contract. There have been many studies that seem to indicate that cancer tends to run in families, but it is not known if there is a genetic component at work here, or if it is because members of a family generally share the same diet, environmental exposure to carcinogens, and so on. (More studies need to be done here, also.)

HORMONES

Hormone levels can have an effect on cancer. Testosterone boosts blood levels   of the bad cholesterol (known as LDL or low-density lipoprotein) and decreases levels of the good one (HDL or high-density lipoprotein), increasing the risk for heart disease and stroke. Estrogen, on the other hand, has beneficial effects on cardiovascular health, lowering LDL cholesterol and increasing HDL cholesterol. A University of Washington study found that estrogen produces these effects by regulating the activity of liver enzymes involved in cholesterol metabolism. Estrogen is an antioxidant–i.e., it neutralizes free radicals. Estrogen given to a woman after menopause decreases her risk of dying from heart disease and stroke, and helps delay the onset of Alzheimer's disease. One risk factor for cancer is early menarche (the beginning of menstruation).

Another risk factor is late childbirth, or the age at which a woman's first child is born. Women who never have children are at a much higher risk of cancers of the sexual organs.

We know that drugs that interfere with estrogen's effect on the body can prevent breast cancer. This is exactly how drugs like tamoxifen and the osteoporosis drug raloxifene work, and how foods like soybeans are believed to prevent breast cancer. (Please see Chapter Three for more information about soybeans and phytoestrogens, which are plant-based sex hormones.)

Diethyl stilbesterol (DES), which is an artificial female hormone sometimes given to woman to relieve menopausal symptoms, causes cervical and vaginal cancer.

There is a hormonal component to prostate cancer, too. High levels of DHT, or dihydrotestosterone, have been found in men who have prostate cancer. Testosterone is converted by the enzyme alpha-reductase to DHT.

Alcohol alters the levels of certain sex hormones, primarily in the liver, by converting testosterone to estrogen. Sugar can be converted to estrogen by bacteria in the stomach; this is another way that sweets cause obesity–besides being an "empty calorie" food that causes overeating to compensate for the lack of nutrition in foods that are high in sugar, estrogen increases fat in the body, whereas testosterone increases muscle.

Consuming fat increases estrogen levels in the body, while

eating meat, or muscle tissue, increases testosterone levels in the body. This may be one reason why eating large quantities of red meat has been associated with an increased risk of cancer–by increasing the formation of dihydrotestosterone.

ONCOGENES — genes that can turn cancer on and off

Oncogenes are a relatively recent discovery in the field of cancer research, and there was great hope at one time that they would provide a way to cure cancer.

Oncogenes have been found in every cell in our body and in the bodies of all other living organisms, too. They seem to underscore the fact that cancer is an inextricable part of life, and that there must be a reason for cancer to exist. (We'll tell you what that reason is in Chapter Nine.) Initially, it was thought that there was only one type of oncogene, and all we had to do was understand how it worked, and then discover how to turn it off. But then scientists discovered that there were two types of oncogenes: One to turn the cancer on, and one to turn it off, called the "anti-oncogene," which actually turns cancer on when it is lost or inactivated. It was then found that oncogenes can mutate into new types of oncogenes, so even if we had a drug that worked against one type, the oncogene could change into another type, rendering the drug ineffective. And it was hoped that there would be only one oncogene per type of cancer, but it was soon discovered that this was not the case. Over 100 oncogenes have been discovered so far, but, unfortunately, each type of cancer doesn't have its own type of oncogene. In Chapter Seven, we'll tell you exactly where these oncogenes come from and how they fit into our theory on the origin of cancer.

RADIATION

We have all heard the admonition to stay out of the sun to avoid skin cancer, but why does the sun cause cancer? What possible connection could life-giving sunlight have with cancer? We'll tell you what that connection is in Chapter Seven.

SEDENTARY LIFESTYLES

Many studies have shown that a lack of exercise is a risk factor for cancer. The exact mechanism for why this should be true is not known, but it is believed that exercise improves the uptake of oxygen by the cells of the body and speeds up the elimination of wastes by improving the functioning of the cardiovascular system. Physical activity also reduces the amount of circulating LDL cholesterol, the so-called "bad" cholesterol, and lowers the levels of estrogen in women and testosterone in men. All of these factors and more are probably why exercise reduces the risk for cancer.

SMOKING

Smoking is a well-known risk factor for cancers of all kinds (not just lung cancer). There are approximately forty-three known carcinogens in cigarette smoke. The latest studies show that the lung cancer risk ranges from four times higher for Asian-American smokers to twenty to forty times higher for African-American smokers over non-smokers.

VIRUSES

Cat owners are familiar with a disease that their pets can contract called feline leukemia, which is caused by a virus. Other viruses and the cancers they cause are:

Virus	Type of Cancer
Epstein-Barr virus (also causes mononucleosis)	Pharyngeal cancer, Non-Hodgkin's Lymphoma
Helicobacter pylori* (also causes ulcers)	Stomach cancer
Hepatitis B	Liver cancer
HIV (Human Immunodeficiency Virus)	Lymphoma, Kaposi's Sarcoma
Papillomavirus	Cervical cancer

* actually, this is a bacterium

Why do viruses cause cancer? How can they possibly be related to other causes of cancer like chemicals or radiation? There will be more on this relationship in Chapter Seven.

WHAT ARE VIRUSES?

Scientists think that viruses evolved from bacteria that had nearly everything stripped away from them except their RNA or DNA and their outer coating or shell. (This theory on the evolution of viruses fits in perfectly with our theory on the origin of cancer, as we will explain in Chapter Seven.) Viruses evolved a survival strategy of "less is more," i.e., they chose a strategy of trimming down so they could move and reproduce fast. They also possess the ability to form spores and enter a dormant stage when conditions around them are less than favorable for them. These spores are crystalline in nature and are able to withstand extremes of temperature and survive exposure to extremely high levels of radiation; in fact, viruses can even withstand the rigors of travel in outer space. In many respects, viruses seem to be a transition stage between organic matter and inorganic matter, or between the living and non-living. Because there are two types of viruses, RNA and DNA viruses, and RNA is a simpler molecule than DNA, some scientists think that viruses evolved first, before bacteria.

Viruses replicate themselves by finding plant, animal, or bacterial cells, then attaching themselves to the surfaces of these cells and injecting their RNA or DNA into the interior of the cells. This RNA or DNA then attacks the host cell's RNA or DNA and converts it into a miniature virus factory, which churns out copies of the virus. The cells then usually disintegrate and release copies of the virus into the organism at large to infect more cells in that organism, or into the surrounding environment to infect other nearby organisms.

A COMMON THREAD?

Is there a common thread that runs through all of these diverse causes of cancer ?

We're convinced there is, and we'll tell you what that common thread is in Chapter Seven.

SUMMARY

Carcinogens are everywhere. They exist in our bodies and in our environment. They cannot be legislated out of existence.

The only hope we have then is to avoid the obvious carcinogens like smoking, too much sun, too much meat, etc., and try to keep our immune systems strong throughout our lives.

Cancer seems to be reversible. Some cancers, like some forms of leukemia, seem to be fairly easy to cure.

The basic causes of cancer can be grouped into three categories: chemicals, radiation, and viruses.

There is a common thread that runs through all three categories. We'll explain what that common thread is in a later chapter.

CHAPTER 3

THE PREVENTION OF CANCER

It is often hard to discern from what we see and hear in the media exactly what course of action we should take to prevent cancer. We hear so much contradictory advice from scientists and so-called experts that it's hard to know whom to believe. And as scientists learn more about cancer, their advice changes. Here's a good example of this:

From Reuters, April 14, 2002:

Smoking may prevent breast cancer

"Washington (Reuters) - Smoking, one of the biggest causes of cancer and heart disease, may actually help reduce the risk of breast cancer in some women, researchers said Tuesday.

"The finding both surprised and dismayed the international team of scientists who did the study, but they said it may shed light on some of the mechanisms behind breast cancer.

'We would hate it if women started smoking because of this study,' Dr. Paul Kleiheus of the World Health Organization, which helped sponsor the study, said in a telephone interview.

"The study found that smoking reduces by 50 percent the risk of developing breast cancer in women who have a rare genetic mutation that can lead to the disease. The mutation, in the genes BRCA1 and BRCA2, affects on average one in 250 women.

"Kleiheus, who directs WHO's International Agency for Research on Cancer, and colleagues were checking for a variety of lifestyle factors that could affect women with the mutation. It is known that just having a 'bad' gene does not guarantee disease– outside factors count, too. "So they were looking for which factors these might be, and surveyed more than 300 women in the United States and Canada who had BRCA1 or BRCA2 mutations. Half, 186 of them, had developed cancer and half had not. "They asked them about various factors, such as when they had children, what they ate–and whether they smoked.

"The first thing that jumped out at the researchers was the clear link to smoking. 'It was a surprise that smoking was the most striking result,' Kleiheus said.

"'We are a little bit embarrassed,' said Gilbert Lenoir, a biologist at the IARC, who also worked on the study, published in the Journal of the National Cancer Institute.

"'We are embarrassed because we feel that the tobacco industry may propagate this without being responsible.'

"The researchers point out that many more women in industrialized countries such as the United States die from lung cancer than die from breast cancer.

"The American Cancer Society predicts that 80,000 women will develop lung cancer this year and 67,000 will die from it, as compared to 43,500 deaths from breast cancer.

"'I think it wouldn't be a good idea to take up the habit,' Kleiheus said. 'But on the other hand it is important for us, for the scientific community, and for the families that we have some hope for new research to try to come to some preventative measure.'

"The researchers think there is probably a clear mechanism for explaining why smoking has this effect, and they hope that drugs can emulate the effect.

"'If you can inhibit the breast cancer risk in these woman by smoking, then you can also do it by other ways,' Kleiheus said. 'We believe the most likely mechanism is a down-regulation of estrogen metabolism,' he added. 'This is a known effect of smoking.'

"In other words, something in tobacco smoke slows down the breakdown of the female hormone estrogen in the body. Breast cancer is known to be linked to estrogen.

"Kleiheus said perhaps drugs that interfere with estrogen could be developed to prevent breast cancer.

"In fact, they have. Researchers this week said two drugs, the established cancer drug Tamoxifen and the osteoporosis drug Raloxifene, sold as Evista, can prevent breast cancer in women.

"Both interfere with the way estrogen is used by the body.

"Kleiheus said the drugs would have to be tested specifically on women with the BRCA1 and BRCA2 mutations to see if they also worked in this group.

"'Indeed they may be the drugs of choice, but we don't know this at the moment because no study was done with these two agents in this high-risk population,' he said."

The article above seems to suggest that smoking can actually prevent breast cancer in some women. Apparently cigarette smoke contains a substance that causes a reduction in the uptake of estrogen by breast cells. (This is how phytoestrogens or plant estrogens can reduce the growth of breast cancer cells.) With so much contradictory and confusing information out there, it is no wonder that most people just throw up their hands and go on eating and living the way they've always done.

In this chapter, we will present the latest information that scientists have on preventing cancer. Unfortunately, scientists and researchers don't completely explain why these factors prevent cancer, but, in Chapter Eight, we'll tell you why these factors prevent cancer from the perspective of our theory on the origin of cancer.

FREE RADICALS

Most people have heard that free radicals cause cancer. But what exactly are free radicals? Oxygen free radicals are oxygen molecules that are deficient in electrons. They are generated as a by-product of oxygen-based metabolism. Ideally, oxygen and other molecules keep their electrons in pairs. Free radicals create electron pairs by stealing electrons from other molecules, damaging them in the process.

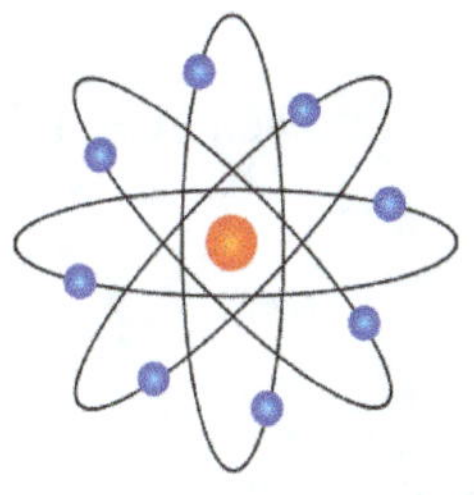

Electrons orbiting around the nucleus of an atom

Antioxidants work by giving up their electrons to stabilize free radicals and prevent them from damaging DNA and other parts of the cell. The most potent antioxidants are vitamins, such as vitamins C and E, provitamins (or precursors to vitamin A, such as beta-carotene), elements such as selenium and zinc, and enzymes such as superoxide dismutase and glutathione.

After decades of research, scientists have found many factors that seem to prevent cancer. Here are a few of those factors:

VITAMINS

Vitamin A, Betacarotene

There have been recent studies that suggest taking betacarotene supplements actually causes a slight increase in mortality from lung cancer. Despite this finding, we still feel that taking higher doses of betacarotene is a good idea, but we recommend that it be taken in the form of vegetables and fruits, such as carrots, squash, tomatoes, alfalfa sprouts, kale, rhubarb, parsnips, yams, sweet

potatoes, broccoli, and seaweed (*nori* and *kombu*, in
Japanese).

Vitamin C

Perhaps the most common vitamin deficiency in the U.S.,
the good news is that this vitamin is easily obtainable from
citrus fruits, such as oranges, lemons, limes; and
vegetables, such as peppers and tomatoes. The bad news is
that we are becoming more and more deficient in this
vitamin, as we consume more prepared, cooked, and fast
foods.
Vitamin C works to prevent free radical formation by
absorbing the energy that creates free radicals. In a later
chapter, we will explain why free radicals cause cancer.

Vitamin D

Vitamin D and calcium work together in our bodies to
prevent skin cancer and colon cancer. Vitamin D is a
protective vitamin that is naturally produced in the skin by
sunlight. When our bodies are deprived of natural light,
our skin produces less vitamin D and less calcium,
resulting in more osteoporosis, especially in women, who
have smaller and thinner bones. There is a constant give-
and-take occurring in our bodies between the calcium in
our bones and the calcium in our blood. Calcium regulates
muscle contraction and is important for the proper
functioning of our heart (hence, the use of calcium channel
blockers in heart disease).

Vitamin E

Another important antioxidant is vitamin E. This vitamin is soluble in oil and prevents the spoiling or oxidation of oil- or fat-based substances in our bodies. It especially protects the lipids in cell membranes from free radical damage. Vitamin E enhances the functioning of the body's immune system and prevents the formation of nitrosamines from nitrites in the stomach. In recent studies in Italy and Finland, it has been shown that higher vitamin E levels in the blood, along with higher levels of other vitamins, reduce the rates of breast cancer and other cancers.

DRUGS

Taxol, Tamoxifen (a cholesterol-lowering drug)

Cancer researchers discovered in the 1940s that certain breast cancer patients did better if they had their ovaries removed. From this, they deduced that certain types of breast cancer were affected by the levels of estrogen in the body.

In the 1960s, researchers discovered that breast cancer cells had receptors on their surfaces that attracted estrogen and induced the breast cancer cells to grow.

Pharmaceutical companies then began developing drugs known as anti-estrogens to treat breast cancer. In the mid-1970s, they created tamoxifen–an anti-estrogen compound that acts like a false estrogen. It took until just recently, however, for these researchers to understand more about

how tamoxifen and other similar drugs work, by acting
like a fake "key" at receptor sites on breast cells and
blocking real estrogen molecules from attaching to these
sites. (In Chapter Eight, we'll explain more about how and
why tamoxifen works to treat and prevent cancer.)

Cis-platinum (Cisplatin)

Cisplatin binds to parts of DNA and interferes with the
dividing of cells. This drug relies on the mechanism in the
body to detect faulty cells that eventually causes these
cells to die (called "apoptosis"). Cisplatin is especially
effective in the treatment of testicular cancer. In Chapter
Six, we will discuss how our theory on the origin of cancer
explains how and why cisplatin works against cancer.

Methotrexate

Methotrexate belongs to a group of drugs known as
antimetabolites. These drugs are used to treat cancers of
the breast, head and neck, lung, blood, bone, lymph, and
uterus (and are also effective against psoriasis and
rheumatoid arthritis). This drug works by blocking the
action of an enzyme known as dihydrofolate reductase in
cells that are cancerous (or in skin cells with psoriasis).
Unfortunately, other cells are affected by methotrexate, so
serious side effects, such as hair loss, loss of appetite,
blurred vision and dizziness can occur.

5-fluorouracil and similar drugs

The family of drugs represented by 5-fluorouracil works
by interfering with the process of meiosis (DNA division)

in the cell. Since some cancer cells are among those that divide most rapidly, these drugs work against these forms of cancer. Unfortunately, stomach cells and hair follicles are also among those cells that divide most rapidly, which is why cancer patients receiving these drugs usually become nauseous and lose their hair.

FOODS

Chlorophyll

This green coloring matter in plants is essential to the production of carbohydrates by photosynthesis. Chlorophyll also works to soak up the energy of UV and ionizing radiation and prevent the formation of free radicals.

Indoles, illudin (mushrooms), diallyl disulphide (garlic, onions, chives)

Mushrooms contain illudin, which has antitumor activity against certain kinds of leukemia cells and other cancer cells. Garlic, onion, chives and their relatives contain a chemical called diallyl disulphide, which can inhibit the growth of molds and bacteria. Diallyl disulphide has also been found to be effective at preventing colorectal cancer.

Lactobacilli (miso soup, yogurt), Tuberculosis bacillus, E. Coli

Some scientists have made the observation that some bacteria, such as E. coli, the tuberculosis bacillus, and lactobacilli, seem to kill cancer cells or prevent cancer. We'll explain why this is possible.

Phytoestrogens (plant estrogens)

Soy beans contain phytoestrogens that replace the body's own estrogens, protecting against breast and ovarian cancers. Soy beans also contain genistein, which blocks the supply of blood to tumors.

Sulforaphane (broccoli)

Broccoli and other cruciferous vegetables contain a substance called sulforaphane, which kills the Helicobacter pylori bacterium. This bacterium causes stomach ulcers and is believed to cause stomach cancer.

RADIATION

Natural (visible) light; UV, and Ionizing Radiation (Gamma, X-Ray, Cosmic)

Ultraviolet and ionizing radiation damages DNA and induces carcinogenesis. In experiments with fish DNA, DNA damaged by UV radiation can be repaired by exposure to visible light. In Chapter Seven, we will explain the significance of these findings.

MISCELLANEOUS PREVENTIVE FACTORS

Heat, hyperthermia

It was believed at one time by some scientists that increasing the body temperature of cancer patients could slow down the progression of their disease. In a later chapter, we'll explain why this phenomenon was observed

and why it could possibly work, from the perspective of
our theory on the origin of cancer.

Exercise

Many studies have shown that exercise seems to help slow
the progression of cancer. We'll provide an explanation
for this, too, in a later chapter.

SUMMARY

Free radicals are oxygen and other molecules that are
deficient in electrons. They are thought to damage DNA
and cause cancer. Vitamins, chlorophyll, selenium, and
other substances prevent the formation of free radicals.

Vitamins are fat- or water-soluble organic substances
obtained from plant and animal foods that are essential in
small amounts for normal growth and functioning of the
body. As mentioned above, vitamins prevent the formation
of free radicals and mitigate the damage they cause to
DNA.

Taxol (tamoxifen) is a drug developed from the toxin of
certain types of yew trees that kills tumor cells.

Cis-platinum (Cisplatin) is an anti-cancer agent whose
development began in the 1960's by accident. During an
experiment with bacteria in electrical fields, it was noticed
that the bacteria stopped multiplying when something
started leaching out of the electrodes. The substance was
identified as platinum.

Methotrexate and 5-fluorouracil are antimetabolites that work by blocking enzymes that cancer cells need to live.

Alkylating agents are a family of anticancer drugs that interfere with the cell's process of division and inhibit cancer cell growth.

Chlorophyll works to prevent cancer by reducing the formation of free radicals, especially by ultraviolet radiation.

Indoles, illudin, and diallyl disulphide are found in cruciferous (cabbage-family) vegetables, mushrooms, and garlic and onions respectively. They have anti-cancer properties.

Lactobacillus is found in fermented foods, such as miso and yogurt, and is thought to prevent cancer.

Phytoestrogens block the action of regular estrogens. Estrogen can promote the growth of breast cancer cells.

Natural light can reverse the DNA damage caused by UV radiation.

Heat or hyperthermia was thought to have anti-cancer activity at one time.

CHAPTER 4

THE ORIGIN OF LIFE

There are two schools of thought concerning the origin of life on the Earth, one that includes divine intervention and one that doesn't. Since we are concerned with the latter, we'll explain scientists' best guesses on how life originated on this planet based on their studies of DNA, bacteria and viruses, the geological and fossil record, and the sciences of astronomy and cosmology (the origin of the universe and our solar system). We will discuss the timeline for the origin of life on this planet and show where the origin of cancer falls on that timeline.

One of the most important questions that scientists are concerned with is why life originated in the first place. There is one school of thought holding that life naturally occurs from non-life and that inanimate matter naturally organizes itself into the basic building blocks of life. Some proponents of this theory contend that life probably originated extraterrestrially, on Mars, for example, but died out at an early stage (or possibly went underground) and that it may be originating on Europa, one of the moons of Jupiter, even now. Some scientists believe that life may have originated more than once on Earth, but that comets and asteroids colliding with the Earth, which occurred much more frequently when the Earth was young, repeatedly wiped out all traces of life. It was only when these collision events became much rarer that life could establish a foothold on the Earth. And when scientists examine the fossil record, it appears that life began almost without hesitation, as soon as it was safe to do so.

Scientists estimate that the Earth originated about 4.6 billion years ago, but heat and radiation levels were too high for life to flourish until about 3.8 billion years ago. The first fossil traces of bacteria are thought to be about 3.5 billion years old and are similar to present-day cyanobacteria (see the section on stromatolites below).

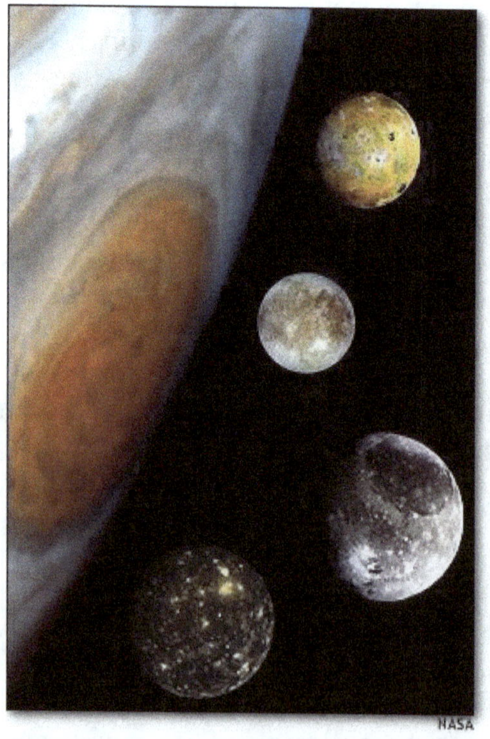

Photo: Europa (second from the top) and the other large moons of Jupiter with a close-up of the giant red spot. (NASA Photo)

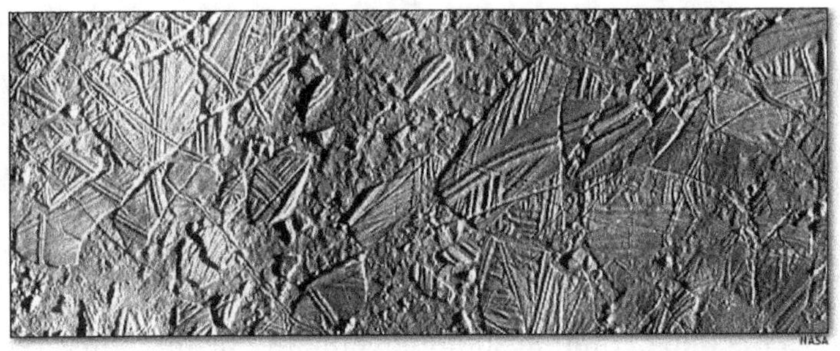

Photo above: Europa's surface, taken by the Galileo space probe launched in 1989, shows an icy crust that has been repeatedly fractured and healed. (Jet Propulsion Laboratory, Caltech Photo)

Some scientists believe that inanimate chemicals can't help but organize themselves into cells, or what could be called "pre-cells," which are more like bubbles or simple structures with membranes. The development of a cell with a membrane was a crucial prerequisite in the origin of life, because a membrane keeps the contents of the cell from dissipating into the surrounding environment. When scientists examined how bubbles and membranes form, they discovered that chemicals seem to want to form these structures. Nobody yet knows why this is so.

It is also not known why nature seems to progress from simple molecules to more complex ones. It is obvious that both nature and humans seem to naturally evolve from simpler forms of organization to more complex ones. But scientists don't know the exact reasons why this should be so.

Another mystery is why certain species of animals and plants remain unchanged for millennia and others evolve into something else, except for the phenomenon called natural selection. Natural selection works to weed out less successful species and rewards the more adaptable and resilient. But it is not clearly understood why there are now both simple organisms and more complex ones; it seems like evolution should eventually result in just complex organisms, especially after four billion years. But life on this planet would not be possible, of course, without the simpler organisms, because they recycle nearly all of the basic requirements of life.

A requirement for a cell to be living is for it to absorb nutrients, use energy, and produce wastes. A cell can produce its energy in a number of different ways: through fermentation[6] (without the use of oxygen), through glycolysis7, and through aerobic metabolism (using oxygen), which is how we derive our energy. Each method is increasingly more complex and parallels the evolution of the planet's atmosphere from a "reducing" one (high in hydrogen compounds) to an "oxidizing" one (which contains a large quantity of free oxygen).

Another requirement for life is the ability to reproduce through some molecule such as RNA or DNA. Some scientists now think that DNA originated from the simpler RNA molecule, which, in turn, originated from a simple spirochaete-like bacterium.

These spirochaete-like bacteria are thought to be responsible for the dance-like mitosis, or fissioning of the cell into two cells, where before there was only one cell.

Here is the current thinking on the timeline for the origin and evolution of life on Earth, and when we believe cancer originated. The supporting evidence for our theory on the origin of cancer can be found in the next chapter:

THE CHRONOLOGY OF LIFE AND THE ORIGIN OF CANCER

TIME   EVENT

13.7 billion years ago   Big Bang

4.5 billion years ago   Earth forms

4.2 billion years ago   Earth cools—
atmosphere: methane (CH_4), ammonia (NH_3), hydrogen, water

4.0 billion years ago   Origin of life—
progenotes, anaerobic fermentation begins, Archaebacteria evolve; secondary atmosphere forms: water vapor, carbon dioxide (CO_2), carbon monoxide (CO), nitric oxide (NO), nitrogen (N_2), sulfur dioxide (SO_2), hydrochloric acid (HCl)

3.5 billion years ago   Stromatolite-forming organisms evolve (photosynthetic blue-green algae and bacteria evolve); nature invents chlorophyll—photosynthesis begins; endosymbiosis[8] begins

3.2 billion years ago   First fossil evidence of bacteria (anaerobic); chemosynthetic autotrophs (for example, the methane producers), saprophytic heterotrophs (decaying organic matter-eaters), parasitic heterotrophs (which eat other organisms)

Atmosphere slowly changes from reducing (rich in hydrogen-containing compounds like methane) to oxidizing (rich in oxygen) as photosynthesizing organisms increase

Aerobic bacteria evolve (oxygen-using)—respiration begins—facultative aerobic bacteria[8] evolve

"Cancer cells" evolve from facultative aerobic bacteria and, through endosymbiosis, the cells of all subsequent life forms acquire the potential to become cancer cells (see the Synopsis of Our Theory on the Origin of Cancer at the beginning of this document)

1.5 billion years ago   Oxygen level in the atmosphere reaches the present level (about 20%)

1 billion years ago   Eukaryotes (organisms made up of cells with distinct nuclei) evolve— Multicellular organisms evolve (sexual reproduction begins)

500-700 million years ago   Fossil record of more complex organisms begins: worms, sponges, jellyfish, etc.

400 million years ago   First land vegetation (plants) and insects

290 million years ago   First evergreens
(pine trees), ferns, gingkoes– First reptiles

200 million years ago   First dinosaurs
and mammals

70 million years ago   First primates

65 million years ago   Dinosaurs
become extinct

35 million years ago   First apes

4 million years ago   Australopithecus
afarensis (human predecessor)

2.5 million years ago   Homo habilis
(more recent human ancestor)

1.5 million years ago   Homo erectus

140,000 years ago   Early Homo
sapiens (our species)

POTASSIUM-ARGON DATING, CARBON-14 DATING

How is it possible to know with any degree of certainty
how old a rock or fossil is? How can scientists be so sure
when they say that the oldest rocks on Earth are 3.8 billion
years old? Scientists believe that all elements on Earth,
such as carbon, gold, silver, uranium, oxygen, and so on
were formed in a supernova billions of years ago. A

supernova is created when much of the material in a star explodes, resulting in an extremely bright, short-lived celestial object, which emits enormous amounts of energy.

Over time, all of these elements decay and gradually change into simpler elements on the Periodic Table. This is what happens to potassium, too. A beta particle[10] hits a proton in the potassium atom and converts it into a neutron, transforming the potassium atom into an argon atom. (Argon is a Noble gas, which is a much more stable element.) This process occurs at a known rate, which is in the millions of years. Scientists can measure the ratio of potassium and argon in a rock sample or fossil with very sensitive scientific instruments and calculate fairly accurately how old that sample is.

Carbon-14 dating works in a similar way, but its time scale is in the thousands of years, instead of in the hundreds of millions of years. Carbon-14 dating is used for much more recent artifacts and fossils.

———————————————

THE BIG BANG

We've all heard astronomers and others talk about the Big Bang, which is the prevailing theory on the origin of the universe. It is based on the observation made by astronomers that the universe appears to be expanding and that the farther out you look with the most powerful telescopes on Earth and in space, the faster the galaxies and stars seem to be receding or moving away from us. By working backwards from the present locations of these galaxies and stars, astronomers have deduced that the universe was created from a massive explosion that occurred at one definite point in the universe about fifteen billion years ago–hence, the name Big Bang. All of the galaxies, stars, planets, the Earth, and all life on this planet, including humans, were created from this explosion.

About four and a half billion years ago, the Solar System formed from a spinning cloud of hot dust and other star stuff. The early Earth had little or no oxygen in its atmosphere at that time, because this was before the evolution and rise of photosynthetic organisms, which throw off oxygen as a waste by-product of their metabolism. As a result, there was no protective ozone layer in the upper atmosphere and the surface of the Earth was under constant bombardment by ultraviolet, gamma, and other forms of radiation from the sun. At the same time, the young Earth was under a constant barrage of asteroids and comets, some large enough to cause devastation on a global scale. (These collisions would result in the mass extinctions of many life forms later in Earth's history.) Volcanic eruptions, too, were occurring much more frequently on the surface of the early Earth at this time.

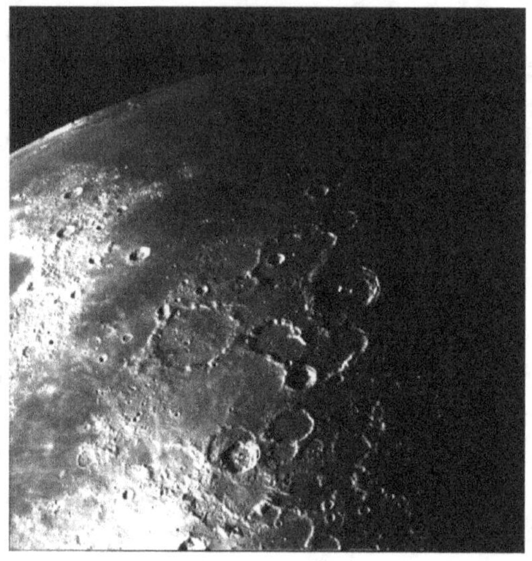

View of the Moon's north polar region

The moon, too, has been hit by many celestial objects, such as comets, meteors, and asteroids. In the photo above, you can see many craters and whitish areas where the subsurface soil material has been ejected by impacting objects. The same process was and is occurring to the Earth, but because large areas of this planet are covered by oceans and because of wind, rain, and tectonic plate drift, we don't see as many craters on the surface of the Earth.

WHAT ARE COMETS, ASTEROIDS AND METEORITES?

Comets resemble dirty snowballs and are a mixture of ice, pebbles, and rocks. They are generally about a half mile to 100 miles wide. The most famous comet is Halley's Comet, which is visible in the sky every seventy-six years (see the amazing photo of Halley's Comet below).

Asteroids are larger "mini-planets" that are mostly found in the asteroid belt between Mars and Jupiter, which sometimes come within a few hundred thousand miles of the Earth. Some have even hit the Earth in the past, causing widespread devastation and mass extinction of species. Meteorites (also known as "shooting stars") are small pieces of rock or ice that have broken off of asteroids or comets and fallen through the Earth's atmosphere.

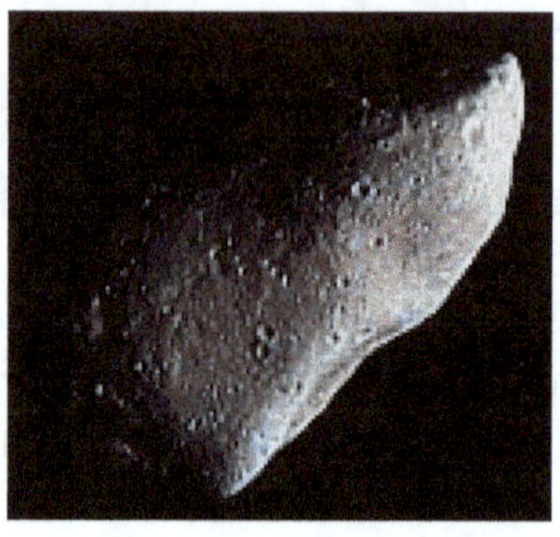

Gaspara asteroid (taken from the
Galileo spacecraft)

An actual photography of
Halley's Comet (from the
Giotto Mission)

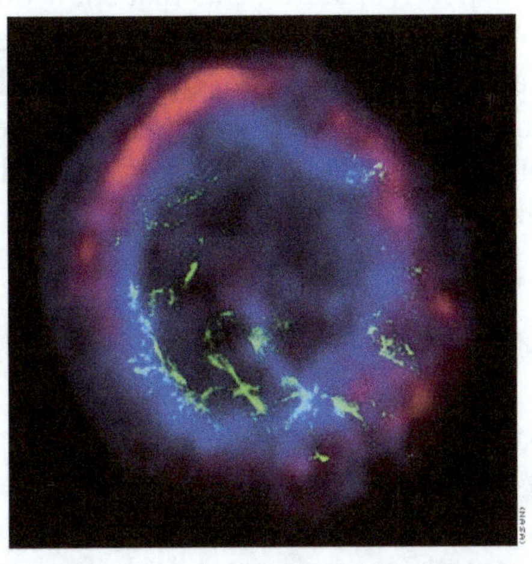

A supernova (NASA false-color photo) –
"We are all star stuff." – Carl Sagan

As the Earth cooled, comets brought organic molecules
such as amino acids (the basic building blocks of proteins)
and enormous quantities of water to the Earth–so much
water, in fact, that the oceans now cover about seventy
percent of the surface. Comets also carry with them such
chemicals as methane and carbon monoxide. When life
first appeared on the Earth four billion years ago, the
number of comets in the vicinity of the sun was hundreds
or thousands of times greater than it is now, so the
quantity of these chemicals must have been quite
substantial.

Some scientists believe that life originated at the bottom of the oceans near volcanic vents that spew out sulfides and other noxious chemicals, safe from the killer radiation of the sun and the raining down of comets and asteroids. From this, these scientists surmise that the earliest life forms on Earth probably had a sulfur-based, non-photosynthetic metabolism.

THE INVENTION OF PHOTOSYNTHESIS

The next great evolutionary leap forward in the history of life was the invention of photosynthesis. As the Earth cooled and water could collect in liquid form and not burn off as steam, there was a great deal of selection pressure on life forms to conquer new frontiers and escape from predators in the volcanic vents, their old stomping grounds.

Living organisms soon developed the means to use water, carbon dioxide, and the energy of the sun to live on. The fortuitous consequence of this was the fact that these life forms produced a waste by-product called oxygen.

Photosynthesis was such a successful invention that there was soon an evolutionary explosion of new organisms that adopted this way of life, and the oxygen level in the atmosphere started to rise precipitously. As the oxygen level rose, the ozone layer formed high in the atmosphere, filtering out much of the damaging UV and other radiation from sunlight (the Earth's magnetic field also helps in this process), making the Earth's surface much more hospitable to life. Because of this new development, life could leave the depths of the oceans and colonize the surface of the Earth. The increasing levels of oxygen in the oceans and atmosphere provided an incentive or selection pressure to use this element for metabolism. The result of using oxygen for metabolism was that about eighteen times as much energy could be derived from a molecule of sugar through oxidation than through fermentation. But because oxygen reacts so readily with other elements–in fact, scientists call oxygen the "Universal Poison"–nature had to invent new chemicals, such as vitamins C and E and superoxide dismutase, to minimize the damaging effects of this gas.

It was around 3 billion years ago that the so-called "red beds" and "Banded Iron Formations" or BIFs appear in the geological record, as the oxygen that photosynthetic organisms released combined with the iron in the Earth's crust to form rust on a global scale. Once nature invented ways to deal with the corrosive effects of oxygen, there was another explosion of new life forms that adopted the aerobic way of life (including us).

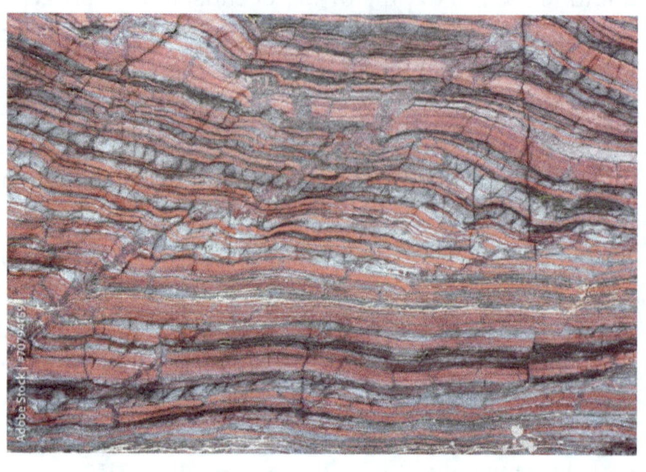

Banded Iron Formations (BIFs)

PROGENOTES

The first life forms on Earth are called progenotes. Progenote is derived from the word progenitor, which means a direct ancestor or precursor. There is still some question as to whether progenotes originated here on Earth, or were brought to Earth by comets or other celestial bodies from elsewhere in the universe (this is called the panspermia theory, which argues that life arrived on Earth from other parts of the universe). Because amino acids and the other building blocks of life have been found in comets, and because bacteria can exist in extremely inhospitable environments such as those in outer space, it has been proposed that life may have been brought to the Earth by comets. Because the underlying basis of metabolism for simple organisms such as bacteria and viruses is inorganic (it is based on the oxidation of iron), some scientists feel that life originates rather readily where even the minimum requirements are met.

Progenotes are RNA-based monera, or single-celled organisms without nuclei.

RNA is a much simpler genetic molecule than DNA, but is still found in the cells of present-day organisms and is used for various cell functions, such as transmitting information from the nucleus to other parts of the cell.

ARCHAEBACTERIA

The Archaebacteria evolved after the progenotes and are a group of ancient bacteria made up of such species as the methanogenic (methane-producing) bacteria, the extreme halophilic bacteria (bacteria that can exist in high-salt environments, such as the Great Salt Lake), and the thermoacidophilic bacteria (bacteria that can exist in high temperatures and highly acidic environments, such as in the geysers of Yellowstone National Park). Archaebacteria differ from other bacteria in the sequence of RNA in their ribosomes (which are tiny protein-synthesizing bodies in the cell), in the absence of muramic acid[12] in their cell walls, and in the lack of glyceryl esters (a type of sugar alcohol) in cell lipids (fats). They appear to be the remnants of a primitive group of organisms that were capable of synthesizing organic compounds before the evolution of photosynthesis.

Evolutionary biologists believe that the original precursor cell was a prokaryotic bacterium like the mycoplasma bacterium. (See the picture above.) Through endosymbiosis[13], this bacteria merged with an aerobic bacteria creating a mitochondria[14]- containing amoeboid-type organism, known as a protista.[15] The aerobic bacteria that became the mitochondria has a modern-day relative, which still exists, called bdellovibrio, an oxygen-using bacterium that invades other bacteria. Scientists are fairly certain that mitochondria evolved from a bacterium that merged with the host bacterium, because mitochondria have their own DNA, which is separate from the DNA in the nucleus. All life forms that evolved after this, including us, have mitochondria, which is inherited only from the mother. Thus, the bacterium that evolved into mitochondria could be considered the "mother (bacteria) of us all."

When the protista merged with a worm-like spirochaete, a more mobile bacterium was created with a whip-like tail that could propel it through its environment. Interestingly, if you slice the tail of this bacteria with a micro-knife, its cross-section would look almost exactly like the tail of a human sperm cell. (More evidence that supports the theory of evolution and the concept of the basic unity of all life on this planet.) The spirochaetes were probably responsible for another important contribution to evolution: it is now believed that they merged even farther into the interior of the cell and became responsible for the phenomenon of mitosis, where the DNA splits and makes an exact copy of itself and forms two identical "daughter" cells.

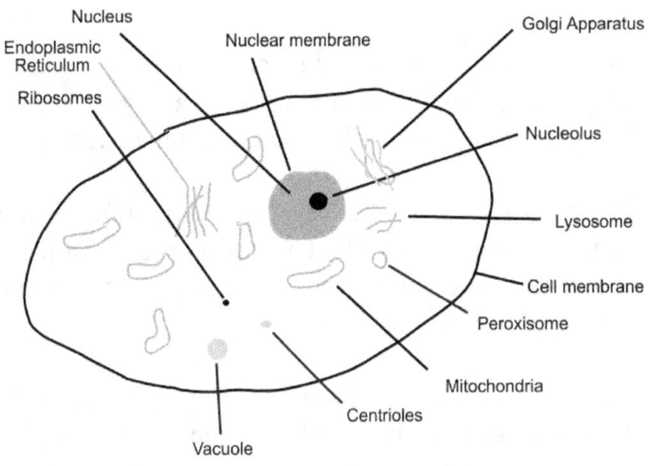

A Typical Cell

When the protista with the whip-like tail joined with a chlorophyll-containing blue-green bacteria, it created the precursor to all plant life on this planet. We can conclude from the fact that plants also develop tumors[16], that the Cancer Cell trait inherited by all subsequent life forms originated before plants and animals diverged on our evolutionary timeline.

CYANOBACTERIA

Cyanobacteria are aquatic and photosynthetic, which means that they live in the water and can manufacture their own food. Because they are bacteria, they are tiny and usually consist of only one cell, although some grow in colonies large enough to see with the naked eye.

Their fossil remains are the oldest known fossils at more than 3.5 billion years old. Cyanobacteria are still around; in fact, they are one of the largest and most important groups of bacteria on Earth.

Many oil deposits are the result of cyanobacteria. They are also important producers of nitrogen fertilizer in the growing of crops like rice and beans. The cyanobacteria have been a tremendously important force in shaping the course of evolution and in ecological change throughout Earth's history; they are responsible for creating the oxygen atmosphere that we depend on. Before they arrived on the scene, the Earth's atmosphere had a very different chemistry, which was inhospitable to life as we know it today, but was ideal for the origin of life.
If it were not for the cyanobacteria, there would not be any plants. The chloroplast inside the cells of plants that allows them to manufacture their own food had its origins as a cyanobacterium that merged into certain eukaryotic[17] bacteria through endosymbiosis.

STROMATOLITES

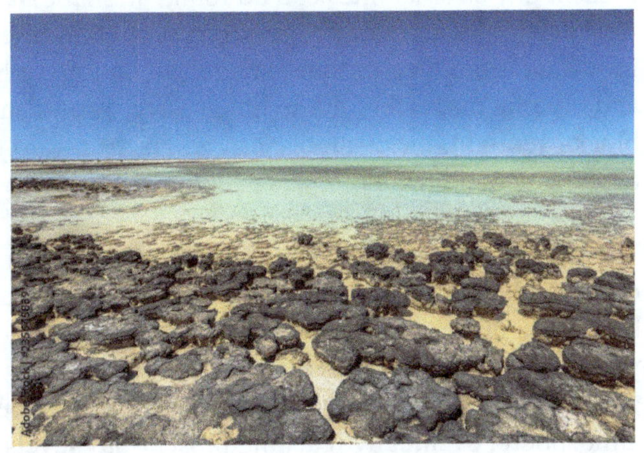

Stromatolites in Shark Bay on the west coast of Australia

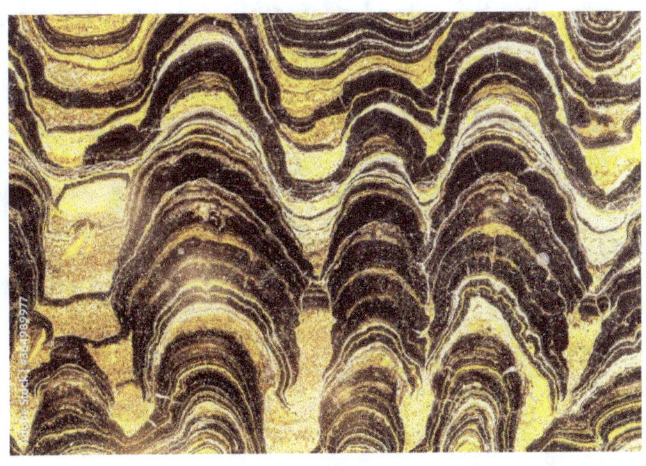

Fossilized Stromatolite

Fossilized stromatolites that are found in certain locations on Earth provide evidence of the earliest cyanobacteria. Present day stromatolites can be found at Shark Bay on the west coast of Australia. Cyanobacteria photosynthesize, grow and reproduce forming layers, which trap sediment and organic matter. As the sediment layer grows and blocks sunlight, the cyanobacteria migrate upward to start a new layer and the old layers eventually fossilize.

The oldest stromatolites are three and a half billion years old, but the stromatolite- forming cyanobacteria really became abundant in the oceans only about 2.3 billion years ago. Photosynthesis by these cyanobacteria generated oxygen, which slowly accumulated in the atmosphere, eventually reaching present-day levels (approximately 21%) by about
billion years ago.

These cyanobacteria are common even today in the oceans, but the domed stromatolite shapes only form in lagoons with highly saline water where larger marine animals don't exist. In parts of the ocean where there are many marine animals, these creatures will eat through the layers so the layers don't survive long enough to form stromatolites.

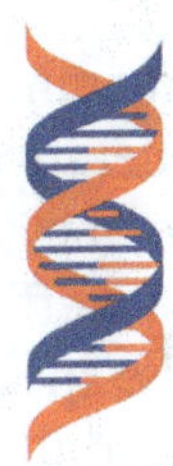

We've all heard about DNA, especially to identify criminals, but what exactly is DNA? DNA is a molecule that consists of a binary (actually, quaternary) code that is similar to the zeroes and ones used to program computers. (In fact, scientists are now using experimental DNA computers to perform computations.) DNA resembles a blueprint which contains the codes for the proteins that make up our bodily structures and enzymes and other biochemicals. The quaternary code consists of the following molecules, which are called nucleotides[18]: adenine (A), thymine (T), cytosine (C), and guanosine (G). One of the rules of DNA formation is that adenine can only bond with thymine, and cytosine can only bond with guanosine. But even with this restriction, there can be millions and millions of different combinations or sequences of nucleotides. In human DNA, there are approximately three billion pairs of A & T and G & C, which are called base pairs, organized into about 30,000 genes.[19] Each combination of three of these base pairs codes for a certain amino acid, which are the basic building blocks of proteins. There are only about twenty amino acids, but, from these amino acids, millions of different proteins can be created.

DNA is found in every living organism from the tiniest viruses to the largest mammals on Earth. It is passed on from generation to generation. Tiny flaws in the sequences can cause mutations; some of these mutations are favorable, some have no effect, and some are damaging to the organism. All of the species that presently exist on the Earth–maybe about ten million in all–and all that have ever existed on the Earth have developed over the last four billion years through these mutations; this may be hard to believe, but there is now a great deal of evidence from microbiology (the study of bacteria and viruses), paleontology (the study of fossils), and molecular genetics (the study of DNA) that supports the theory of evolution.

If you examine the genes of yeast, flies, and worms, you see the same genes in all three species; these genes may not have exactly the same functions in the three species, but they will have similar functions. We humans, too, share genes with the lowly yeast cell. What does this mean? Again, it means that all life is basically one, and all species share a common ancestor.

How do new genes arise? Humans obviously have more complexity than yeast cells and have many more genes. How then are these new genes created? New genes are created by the doubling of old genes with a gradual change in function for the new genes.

WHAT ARE BACTERIA?

Four billion years ago, when bacteria evolved into being, the Earth was a very different place than it is now. There was no free oxygen in the atmosphere, which meant that there was no ozone layer to shield out the deadly radiation from the sun. There were frequent bombardments from meteors, comets, and asteroids, which wiped out any incipient life (probably many times). There were volcanic eruptions that spewed out sulphurous gases and other noxious chemicals, and much more radiation from decaying uranium 235, which was about fifty times more abundant then, in the soil, oceans, and atmosphere, than now. In spite of these hellish conditions on Earth, bacteria thrived and multiplied. New species arose to meet the challenges of different environmental conditions. There were bacteria that flourished in extremely acidic or alkaline environments, or in environments of extreme pressure, such as those found at the bottom of the deepest oceans. Temperature wasn't a problem either; there are bacteria that have been found growing at 112° Celsius (233° Fahrenheit) in geysers deep underground. There are bacteria that can feed on nitrogen, sulphur, and other simple inorganic molecules; they don't require any organic food at all. There are bacteria that can live without sunlight, at the depths of the oceans where undersea geothermal vents provide the sulphurous compounds and the energy that these bacteria need. Certain bacteria can live on oil found in oil deposits miles beneath the surface. There are even some bacteria that can create methane from carbon dioxide and hydrogen and derive energy from this process, then metabolize that methane for more energy, releasing carbon dioxide and hydrogen, in a kind of perpetual motion machine.

Perhaps the most amazing fact about all of this is that all of these different kinds of bacteria still exist today, which is a good thing because we couldn't have developed our theory on the origin of cancer without them.

KEY SOURCES FOR THIS CHAPTER:

For more information on endosymbiosis and the evolution of bacteria and viruses, see these books written by Dorion Sagan and Lynn Margulis (Carl Sagan's son and ex- wife, who was a distinguished professor of biology at the University of Massachusetts in Amherst):

GARDEN OF MICROBIAL DELIGHTS. (1993). Dorion Sagan and Lynn Margulis. Kendal/Hunt Publishing Co.

MICROCOSMOS. (1986). Dorion Sagan and Lynn Margulis. University of California Press. (See especially Chapter 8 in this book.)

THE ORIGIN OF EUKARYOTIC CELLS. (1970). Lynn Margulis. Yale University Press.

SUMMARY

Scientists think that the universe was created about 13.7 billion years ago with the Big Bang.

There are two schools of thought concerning the origin of life on the Earth: the Panspermia theory that says that life originated elsewhere in the universe and was brought to the Earth by celestial bodies, and the other theory that says that life originated natively here on Earth.

The early Earth was a hellish place with many volcanoes and collisions with comets and asteroids. There was no ozone layer to shield the surface from UV-, cosmic-, and gamma-radiation.

The early Earth had a reducing atmosphere high in hydrogen and hydrogen compounds, such as methane, which is toxic to most present-day life, but was perfect for the creation of life.

The first life forms were bacteria and viruses. The evolution of these life forms mirrors the composition of the atmosphere. The rise of the cyanobacteria that lived by photosynthesis produced a toxic byproduct called oxygen. Eventually, so much oxygen was produced that the atmosphere is now about 20% O_2.
The earliest bacteria were the Archaebacteria that could live without oxygen or sunlight, in extremes of temperature and pressure.

The next bacteria to evolve were the eukaryotes, which had distinct nuclei. Some bacteria used endosymbiosis to merge and help each other survive. (In fact, we are all just a collection of these bacteria that merged.)

Metabolism using oxygen produces so much more energy per molecule of food that soon many organisms using this form of metabolism evolved. We are one of them.

CHAPTER 5

WHAT IS EVOLUTION? WHAT IS NATURAL SELECTION?

How is it possible that something as complex and wondrous as a human being could develop from the primordial slime that existed billions of years ago? We are so different from bacteria and viruses that evolution seems impossible. Actually, when we examine the chemistry and structure of human cells, we see that we aren't that different from bacteria and viruses. There are a great many clues to our bacterial origins; for example, the basic homology or structure of our DNA is the same as that of bacteria, and, in fact, this is what makes it possible to identify criminals through DNA testing. We use bacteria to multiply tiny quantities of human DNA to make the characteristic patterns of elongated black dots on paper that help investigators solve crimes. The DNA of humans is folded and wrapped around itself in a pattern that resembles the pattern found in bacterial DNA, and there are large sections of base pairs in our DNA that are the same as the patterns found in the DNA of bacteria and other more complex organisms.

One may think that the basic structure of our bodies, the layout of our arms and legs, and the organization of our organs are different from, say, a worm's, but when you compare the spinal column of humans and the segmented body parts of worms, here, too, you will see many similarities. Again, it is obvious that nature likes to reuse successful inventions over and over again. The cross-section of the tail of a human sperm cell looks identical to the cross-section of the whip-like tails of some bacteria. As a human embryo develops in the womb, it goes through stages that reveal the debt we owe to earlier life forms for the evolution of certain bodily structures. (Scientists call this process, "ontogeny recapitulating phylogeny.") Early in the development of the human fetus, it passes through a stage where it develops what scientists call a notochord, or a piece of cartilage that simple marine animals have in place of a regular backbone. As the human fetus develops further, this notochord becomes a fully-formed backbone. The fetus also briefly exhibits gill plates at one stage in its development; these gill plates eventually become our chin and jaw bones.

The organization of similar groups of bodily structures is controlled by supergenes, which are an important group of genes that are responsible for the supergenes development of the main subsections of the bodies of organisms. Small changes in these can cause very large changes in the physical structure of an organism, and this is how whole new species can develop rather quickly on an evolutionary time scale.

All of these genetic changes are overseen by a process called natural selection, which can best be described as anything that improves the survival advantages of an individual organism or of an entire species. If a change in the internal or external structure or in the behavior of an organism makes it better able to evade predators, find food more efficiently, or find a mate more readily, then this new feature will lead to more offspring with the same trait being produced by that individual. Some of these mutations have the opposite effect and make the organism less likely to survive. These changes are gradually weeded out, and the species as a whole benefits. As the environment changes, those individuals that are most flexible and adaptable to the changes survive and prosper. There can sometimes be an explosion of new species when there is a dramatic change in the environment. This is exactly what happened about 600 million years ago during the Cambrian Era on Earth when the atmosphere began to contain much more oxygen with the rise of photosynthetic organisms. Nature invented aerobic metabolism (metabolism using oxygen) to take advantage of this new development; aerobic metabolism produces much more energy per molecule of food than the old-fashioned anaerobic method of metabolism (i.e., fermentation). Also, around this time, nature invented shells and skeletons made from calcium carbonate. These two new developments sparked a huge increase in the number of new species in what scientists call the "Cambrian Explosion."

Skeptics who feel that evolution could not possibly be responsible for the incredible diversity of life forms on this planet should consider how there are now 400 or so breeds of dogs. All of these breeds have been created through selective breeding from a single wolf-like ancestor in only a few tens of thousands of years. Imagine then if you had billions of years to develop new species, which is exactly what nature had.

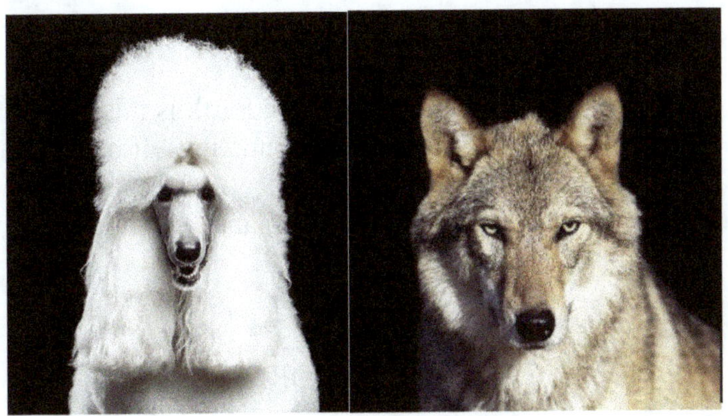

Poodle   Wolf

More evidence supporting evolution is found in the fossil record. For example, as you travel down from the rim of the Grand Canyon to the Colorado River a mile below, you pass through millions of years of sedimentation until you reach rock layers that are more than two billion years old. The fossils in the surrounding sedimentary layers gradually become simpler and simpler until the soil around you at the bottom of the Canyon contains only the fossilized remains of single-celled organisms.

Perhaps the most amazing fact about evolution is that there are now an estimated ten million to one hundred million species of organisms on the Earth. There may be as many as a million different species of bacteria alone. The book, Bergey's Manual of Systematic Bacteriology, lists 4,000 species of bacteria. In a pinch of soil, there are probably about a billion bacterial cells and probably over 10,000 colonies or 8,000 different types of bacteria. In the mouths of human beings, there are about 500 different species of bacteria.

A remarkable fact about life on the Earth is this: the biochemistry involved in the life functions of bacteria and those of all other organisms is basically the same; we humans and all life forms on this planet are truly one.

HOW DOES EVOLUTION WORK?

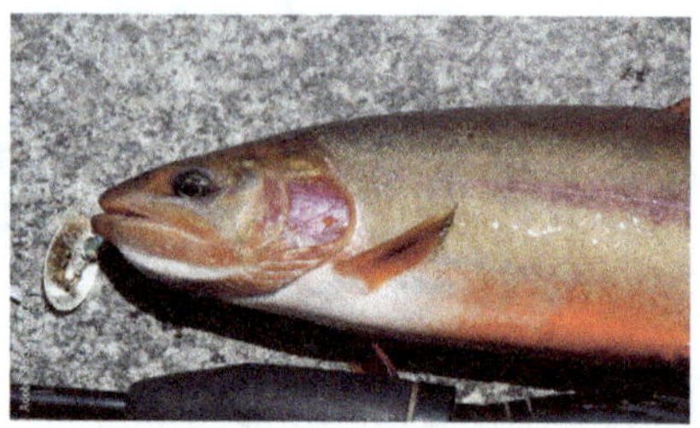

Golden Trout

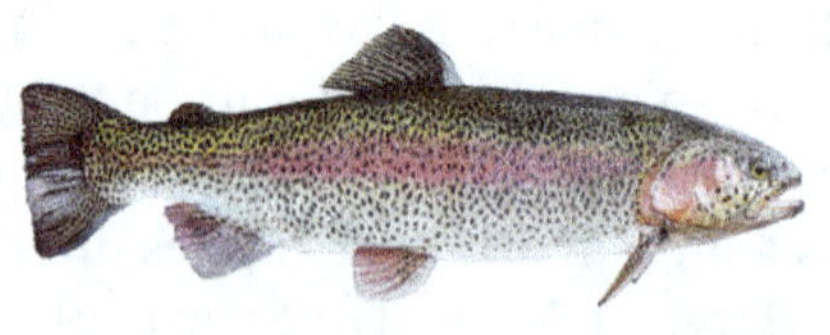

Rainbow Trout

To illustrate how evolution works with one small example, take the case of the Golden Trout, the state fish of California. These beautiful fish are found high in the Sierra Nevada mountains, west of the tiny town of Lone Pine, California. The Golden Trout are descended from the native Rainbow Trout, one of the most popular game fishes in the world.

During a previous Ice Age, the Sierras were covered by large glaciers. As the climate warmed, these glaciers melted and flooded California's Central Valley where the present-day towns of Fresno and Bakersfield are. Ancestral Rainbows, closely related to the Redband Trout, which still exist today in small pockets around the West, came up from the Valley and eventually colonized the streams high in the Sierras via the Kern River. As the climate continued to warm, the lower Kern River dried up and isolated these Rainbows from other Rainbows farther downstream. Eventually, because of different environmental conditions and through intensive interbreeding, these fish took on the spectacular coloring that they now possess.

The Golden Trout has existed as a separate species for only a few tens of thousands of years and can still interbreed with Rainbow Trout. This is an indication that the Golden Trout and the Rainbow Trout share a common ancestor and that they are genetically similar. Given more time, closely-related species like this become more genetically different and soon become unable to interbreed, or if they can interbreed, their offspring are sterile (just like donkeys and horses are bred together to produce mules, which are sterile).

When the same process that created the Golden Trout occurs on a continental scale, we get a whole country full of remarkable animals, such as those found in Australia. The continent of Australia was at one time joined to other continents, but over millions of years, gradually drifted away from them and became isolated. The plants and animals on the Australian continent were able to evolve in "splendid isolation" (as paleontologist George Gaylord Simpson said) from other life forms around the world, which is how such unusual animals as the duck-billed platypus, the kangaroo, and the koala bear developed.

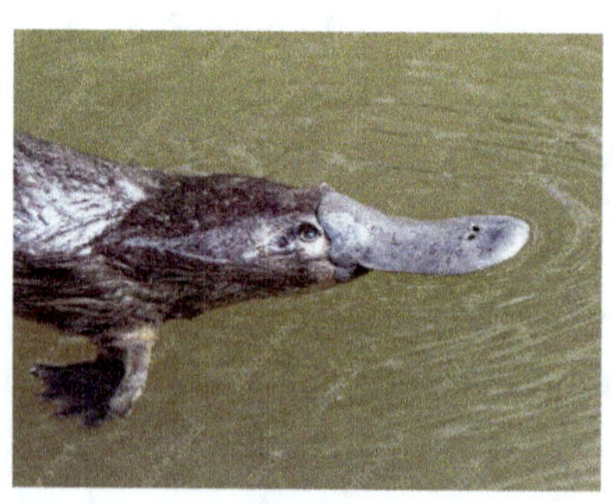

Platypus

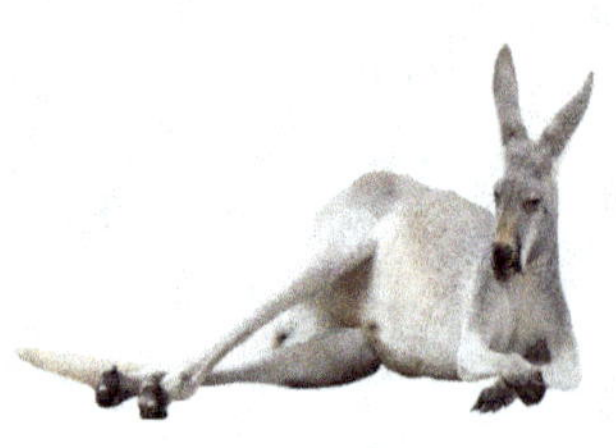

Kangaroo

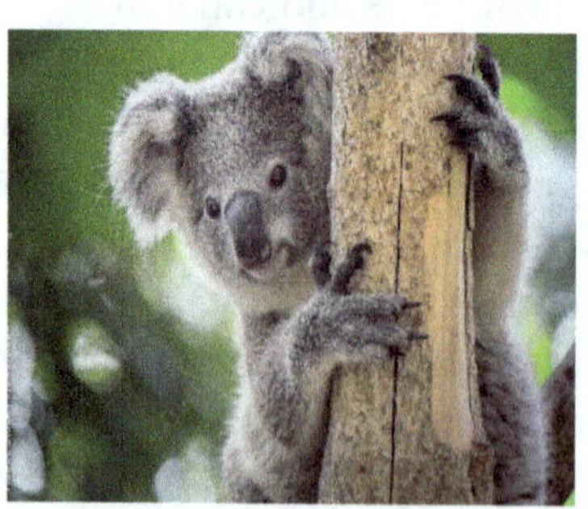

Koala Bear

SUMMARY

The basic shape and chemistry of bacterial DNA and our DNA is the same. There is a unity to all life on this planet.

Nature doesn't reinvent the wheel. It keeps using successful inventions over and over again. For example, the cross-section of the tail of a human sperm cell is identical to that of the tails on some bacteria.

Individual members of species are all slightly different. Mutations in DNA create changes, some of which are good, some are neutral, and others are bad. Mutations that help the animal survive better result in more offspring with that characteristic being produced.

A dramatic change in the environment or a relocation of a species can cause a rapid increase in new species, especially in small, isolated populations. A good example of this on a small scale is the Golden Trout of California, which is derived from the Rainbow Trout. A much larger example is the unusual flora and fauna of Australia.

CHAPTER 6

THE ORIGIN OF CANCER?

THE RIDDLE OF CANCER SOLVED?

Cancer evolved from the methane family of bacteria. Anything that reminds the normal cell of its methanogenic bacterial heritage is carcinogenic–including chemicals, radiation, and viruses.

In September, 1989, we experienced a major epiphany—that it might be useful to study how bacteria and viruses evolved billions of years ago because cancer cells act like bacteria in many ways. (See the section on "HeLa cells" on page 80.) As we learned more about the origin of early life forms, we soon realized that we may have stumbled onto a plausible explanation for how cancer originated.

An important early clue for us about how cancer originated was the picture below, which is from the book, Evolutionary Biology by Douglas J. Futuyma (1986 Sinauer Associates). This drawing of the evolutionary tree of early life forms proved to be a "Rosetta Stone[20]" for us.

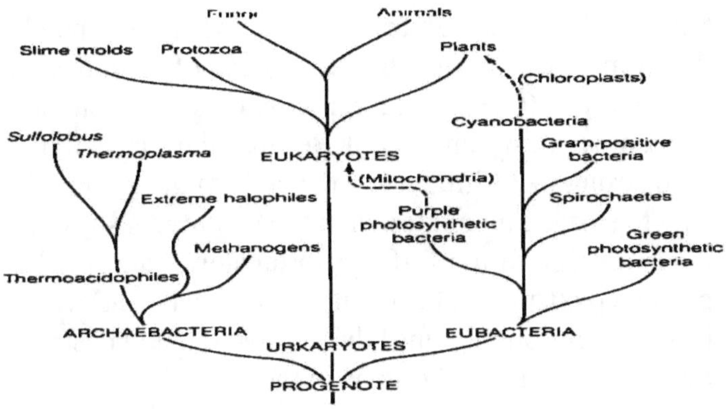

WHY IT IS IMPORTANT TO UNDERSTAND THE ORIGIN OF CANCER

We believe that we will be able to prevent and cure cancer only if we understand how and why cancer originated. Our theory on the origin of cancer explains why normal cells turn cancerous: when cells are under stress, they regress to the way they were when these cells first evolved. A major stressor is when the micro-environment surrounding the cell changes to one favoring a more primitive type of cell, one that, for example, doesn't require oxygen and can exist on fewer nutrients. When this happens, the cell reverts to the "Cancer Cell Way of Life," to a time when early life forms such as bacteria and viruses first originated. This "lifestyle" existed when the Earth was still young, when its atmosphere was full of methane (CH_4), ammonia (NH_3), hydrogen cyanide (HC), ethane (C_2H_6) and other similar gases–much like the present-day atmospheres of other planets in our solar system, such as

Saturn's Titan and Jupiter's Europa, where life may be in the formative stages even now–instead of the nitrogen (N_2), oxygen (O_2), and carbon dioxide (CO_2) that our atmosphere now contains.[21] Because the survival instinct is so strong in all life forms, the cell struggles to find a way to survive no matter what the conditions surrounding it. Cancer is a form of life; unfortunately, cancer cells cannot coexist peacefully with normal cells and want to grow uncontrollably until they crowd out and destroy important tissues and organs in the body. But cancer, too, is the result of natural selection,[22] as we will see in Chapter Nine, so, in a roundabout way, cancer follows the natural law of survival of the fittest. We believe that there might be a survival advantage for cells to retain the Cancer Cell lifestyle, because the environmental conditions that resulted in the origin of cancer and which favor the Cancer Cell lifestyle may return to the Earth again. (See Chapter 9 for more on this.)

HOW THE PROCESS OF ENDOSYMBIOSIS RESULTED IN THE INCORPORATION OF CANCER INTO ALL PLANT AND ANIMAL CELLS

The drawing below contains scientists' best guess on how the major groupings of life forms–bacteria, plants, animals and fungi–evolved along with the evolution of the Earth's atmosphere.

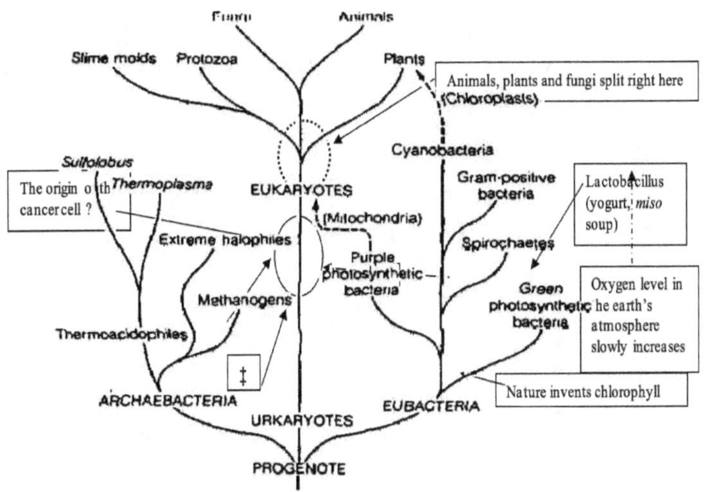

The picture above is the same picture from the book, *Evolutionary Biology*, by Douglas Futuyma we saw earlier in this chapter. We have modified this drawing to show how and when we think cancer originate.

* "Gram-positive" bacteria and the Cancer Cell Prototype Bacteria (i.e., the mycoplasma bacterium) are age-old competitors. They have been rivals for at least three billion years. This would explain why lactobacillus-containing foods, such as yogurt and miso soup[23], are thought to prevent cancer.

‡ The endosymbiosis[24] of the methylotrophic (methane-oxidizing) bacteria and the halophilic (salt-loving) bacteria into the first eukaryotic bacteria[25]
 is the reason why the "Cancer Cell trait" became incorporated into all species of plants26 and animals that subsequently evolve. This may explain why methane-

containing chemicals cause cancer (see chemical carcinogenesis below) and why cancer cells are high in sodium.

DEFINITION OF "GRAM-POSITIVE" AND "GRAM-NEGATIVE":

GRAM-NEGATIVE = stain pink when using dye to make their internal structures visible under the microscope, some practice sex. Examples: *E.coli*, cyanobacteria (asexual); cyanobacteria (anaerobic) practice sex; *rhodopseudomonas*

GRAM-POSITIVE = stain purple, lacks lipoprotein membrane (cholesterol membrane), are asexual, form spores. Examples: *lactobacillus*, *actinomyces*(anaerobes & facultative anaerobes)

GRAM'S STAIN is a method of staining bacterial cells, used as a primary means of identification. A film of bacteria spread onto a glass slide is dried and heat-fixed, stained with a violet dye, treated with decolorizer (e.g., alcohol), and then counterstained with red dye. Gram-negative bacteria lose the initial stain but take up the counterstain, so that they appear red microscopically. Gram-positive bacteria retain the initial stain, appearing violet microscopically. These staining differences are based on variations in the structure of the cell wall in the two groups. [Gram, H. C. J. (1853 - 1938)] - Source: *The Concise Medical Dictionary*. (1998). Oxford University Press/Market House Books Ltd.]

HELA CELLS - NO LONGER HUMAN

Henrietta Lacks was a thirty-year old African-American mother of four who died in October, 1951, of cervical cancer. Cells were taken from her tumor and cultivated in the laboratory. This cell line is still alive today and is widely used in cancer research. Her cell line is called "Helacyton gartleri" after Henrietta Lacks and cytos, which is Greek for cavity or cell, and Stanley Gartler, the geneticist who was the first to document the cells' remarkable longevity. Normal cells are programmed to divide about twenty times and then die. HeLa cells can divide over and over again and are essentially immortal. This is another clue that cancer cells are just like bacteria, which can also divide indefinitely as long as they receive enough nutrients. In fact, we believe that HeLa cells are a very strong clue that normal cells contain the mycoplasma bacterium deep within them.

From *Discover Magazine*, December 1992:

No Longer Human

By Lori Oliwenstein

"HeLa cells came from a human being, but for 40 years now they've been evolving on their own, in petri dishes. They may be a new species.

"Henrietta Lacks achieved a kind of immortality on February 9, 1951. On that day a sample of cancerous cells from her cervix was transferred to a culture dish, doused with nutrients, and left to grow. Lacks, a 30-year-old mother of four from Baltimore, had one of the most aggressive cervical cancers her doctors had ever seen, and the cells culled from her tumor grew avidly, doubling their number each day. Then they escaped. Small spills are always happening in laboratories; what distinguished Lacks's cells was their ability to survive after they were somehow spilled. They were so hardy that if just one of them fell on a petri dish it would outgrow and overwhelm anything else living on that dish within a month.

"Soon Henrietta Lacks's cells were traveling from lab to lab, either deliberately sent–many cancer researchers had taken to using them in their experiments–or as an unseen contaminant tagging along in another cell line. Some researchers who thought they were looking at something completely different–a line of liver cells, say–ended up studying Henrietta Lacks's cervical cells by accident. The cells even slipped through the iron curtain and into Russia.

"Lacks died in October 1951, but her peripatetic cells lived on. Now some biologists are saying that those cells, called HeLa cells for short, have lost more than their connection to Henrietta Lacks. HeLa cells, these researchers claim, are no longer human at all; they are single-celled microbes–closely related to us, to be sure, but their own distinct species.

"How so, you ask? 'HeLa cells are not connected in any way to people,' explains evolutionary biologist Leigh Van Valen of the University of Chicago. 'They have an extremely different ecological niche from us. They don't mate with humans; they probably don't even mate with human cells. They act just like a normal microbial species. They are evolving separately from us, and having a separate evolution is really what a species is all about.'

"The process of evolution is much the same for HeLas as it is for humans, although the former usually reproduce asexually, by cell division. As the cells divide, genetic mutations inevitably occur, and the ones that make the cells better adapted to their ecological niche–the petri dish–are preserved by natural selection. When Henrietta Lacks's cells first became cancerous, they also acquired the ability to survive indefinitely in a culture medium; that massive genetic transformation made them substantially different from ordinary human cells, and after four decades of evolution they have become more different still. Different strains of HeLa cells, analogous to different races of human beings, have even developed in some of the geographically separated lines.

"'These little unicellular organisms have crossed oceans, spread their range, got into other cultures and out competed them,' says Richard Strathmann, a marine biologist at the University of Washington's Friday Harbor Laboratories who dabbles in evolutionary theory. 'They're only different from other single- celled organisms in that a human being gave rise to them.'

"Strathmann and Van Valen (the latter with his colleague Virginia Maiorana) put forth these ideas separately, in two papers in the same issue of the journal Evolutionary Theory, which Van Valen edits. (Both papers, he points out, were independently reviewed before publication.) Van Valen and Maiorana not only declared that HeLa may not be Homo Sapiens, they gave the new species a name: Helacyton Gartleri–Hela, after the HeLa cells themselves; cyton, from the Greek cytos, meaning cavity or cell; and gartleri after geneticist Stanley Gartler, who was the first to document the cells' remarkable success…'"

The article below from the August, 1999 issue of *Discover Magazine* explains how a toxin produced by E. coli kills cancer cells and other bacteria that compete with E. coli.

We think that this is a clue that E. coli and cancer cells co-evolved over three billion years ago.

E. COLI AND CANCER

From *Discover Magazine*, August 1999:

E. Coli Kills Cancer

By Martha Heil

"Cancer is often fought with chemotherapy, and the effects of these toxic drugs can be excruciating. But Canadian researchers have discovered that a familiar, yet potent toxin can actually shrink brain tumors in less than 48 hours with no apparent ill effects.

"The cancer-fighting chemical is verotoxin, which is produced by the ubiquitous E. coli bacteria. This toxin, which causes diarrhea, was injected into human brain tumors implanted in mice. It not only shrank the tumors, but none of the tumors reappeared.

"How can a substance dangerous in the stomach not be dangerous to the brain cells? "What is important is the amount of the toxin," says Dr. Clifford Lingwood of the Hospital for Sick Children in Toronto. Just a little bit of it won't hurt you, but the more you're exposed to, the sicker you'll get. The idea is to find a level that is harmless to the animal as a whole, but deadly to the cancer cells. A study of baboons measured how much verotoxin it would take to make an ape sick. Animals given small doses showed no side effects, nor did the mice in Lingwood's study. "Lingwood says that the verotoxin stops the growth of new blood vessels. "Tumor cells are particularly susceptible," he explains, because the tumors are marked by a specific glycolipid, a receptor that acts as a gateway into the cell.

"The verotoxin finds the glycolipids on tumors and the blood vessels that surround the tumor cells. It attaches itself to the receptor and causes the cells to commit suicide. Verotoxins ignore normal, non-cancerous brain cells, which don't contain the receptor. With the toxin attacking both its outer membrane and its food supply, the brain tumor shrivels almost immediately after treatment begins. In cancer cells in Petri dishes, "You can see a significant difference in 90 minutes," Says Lingwood. "Lingwood's results were reported in the June issue of the journal, Oncology Research. "

The article below discusses other bacterial toxins that can destroy cancer cells.

Novel tumor fighter calls on an unusual mix of allies by Nicholas Wade, New York Times News Service December 21, 2001

"Chemotherapy and radiation are efficient killers of tumor cells, but they are not always effective because many tumors contain central zones devoid of blood and oxygen.

"Drugs cannot reach places where blood does not circulate, and radiation fails in those zones because it needs oxygen to kill cells. The two therapies often let enough cancer cells survive to defeat the treatment.

"A novel method to overcome those obstacles has achieved striking results in mice. Its chief drawback is that the tumors are killed so quickly that their dying cells flood the bloodstream with toxic products, making the cure as bad as the disease for some mice.

"The method was develop by Dr. Bert Vogelstein and colleagues at the Johns Hopkins School of Medicine. Vogelstein is widely known for his work on unraveling the genetics of colon cancer cells, and developing a therapy is a departure from his usual work. He said it would take several years to see if the treatment is suitable for people.

"The therapy has three components–a bacterium that destroys tumors from within, a chemical that attacks cells on the outside of tumors and an agent that makes the tumor's blood vessels collapse.

"Though the potion is rationally designed, its ingredients sound like a witch's brew. The bacterium is a genetically tamed version of Clostridium novyi, a microbe that causes gas gangrene when it gets into wounds.

"The vessel-closing agent, dolastatin-10, was isolated from an Indian Ocean sea hare, Dolabella auricularia, by Dr. George R. Pettit of Arizona State University. And the cell-attacking chemical, mitomycin C, is a poison developed by a soil-dwelling microbe, Streptomyces lavendulae…"

The bacteria mentioned in the article above are Clostridium novyi, a microbe that causes gas gangrene in wounds, and Streptomyces lavendulae, which produces mitomycin C, an antibiotic. The Clostridium novyi microbe can exist only in an anaerobic environment like that which exists in the centers of tumors. We believe that these bacteria kill cancer cells because they are long-time rivals of the mycoplasma bacterium. This is why the antibiotics they produce kill cancer cells, because cancer cells are essentially bacteria; in fact, we believe that they are direct descendants of the methanogenic family of bacteria.

METHANOGENIC BACTERIA

Methanogenic bacteria are a group of archaebacteria (an ancient lineage of bacteria) that produce methane; they include such species as methanobacillus and methanothrix. Methanogens are anaerobic bacteria found in oxygen-deficient environments, such as marshes, swamps, sludge (formed during sewage treatment), and the digestive systems of ruminants like cows and sheep. They obtain their energy by reducing carbon dioxide and oxidizing hydrogen, with the production of methane ($CO_2 + 4H_2 >> CH_4 + 2H_2O$). They utilize chemicals like formate, methanol, and acetate for food and to create their cells. Methanogenic bacteria are important in the production of biogas, which is used by humans for fuel.

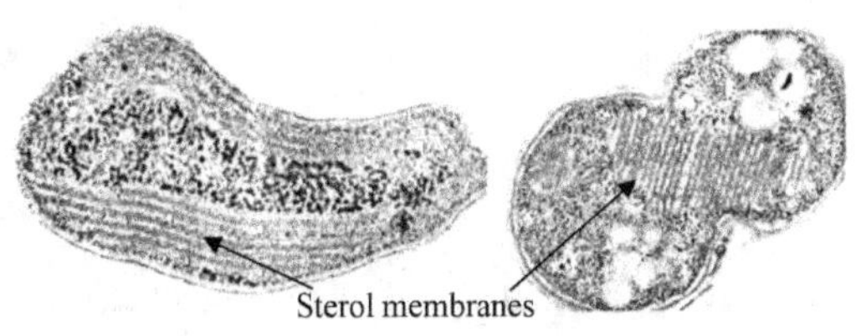

Methanogens

The methanogens were the first bacteria to use sterols to create internal membranes. Sterols were subsequently used by other life forms to create cell membranes, sex hormones, and other substances vital to life. (You can see the ring-like and linear structure of the sterol membranes in the picture of methanogenic bacteria above.) These bacteria evolved before sexual reproduction was invented (and sex hormones had been invented); they reproduce by cloning[27] instead.

PELOMYXA PALUSTRIS

This amoeba offers many clues to the origin of cancer and the incorporation of cancer into the cells of all higher life forms. What makes our work so much easier is that many of the bacteria and other simple organisms that existed billions of years ago still exist today largely unchanged. These organisms provide a detailed step-by-step timeline on how life and the environment on Earth evolved and changed, and help to pinpoint how and when cancer entered the picture.

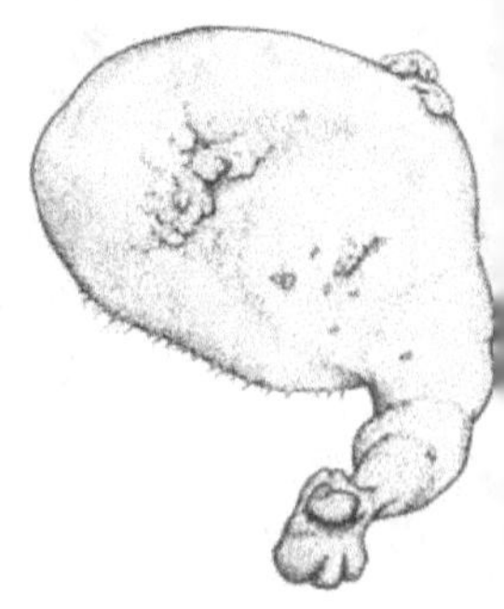

Pelomyxa palustris amoeba

Source: *GARDEN OF MICROBIAL DELIGHTS* by Dorion Sagan & Lynn Margulis. (1993). Kendall/Hunt Publishing Co.

Prokaryote   Eukaryote

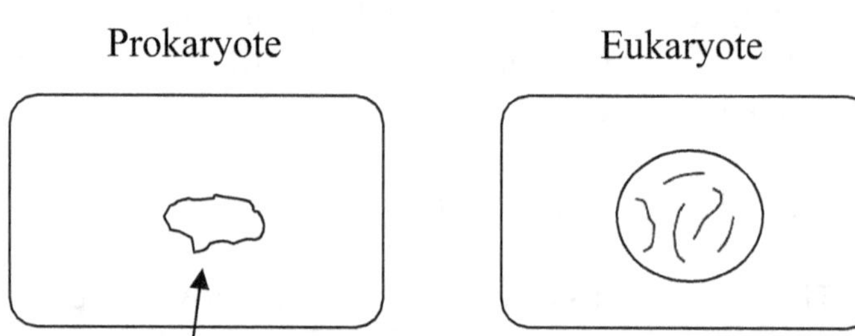

Prokaryotes: Single DNA loop. Has no nucleus.

Eukaryotes: Multiple strips of DNA
Has a distinct nucleus

Prokaryotes vs. Eukaryotes

The Pelomyxa amoeba (see the picture above) is a very unusual and important sole member of the phylum Karyoblastea (i.e., important to our discussion here). It is among the simplest eukaryotic organisms, which means that it was probably one of the first to have a separate and distinct nucleus. This amoeba looks like a wine flask, but is only about 0.5 millimeters long or slightly larger than the period at the end of this sentence. It feeds on one-celled animals and plants, mostly bacteria and algae. It is microaerophilic, which means that it needs only tiny amounts of oxygen to survive (this is an indication that it probably evolved when low-oxygen conditions existed on Earth). Pelomyxa is still found today in freshwater pond scum, where there is usually little or no oxygen. It contains no oxygen-breathing mitochondria; instead, it has three different types of symbiotic bacteria living inside of it: one species lives in neat rings around the nuclei (of which it has many–just like some cancer cells28); another species metabolizes lactic acid, a waste product generated by the Pelomyxa itself and which would eventually kill it if this chemical were not consumed; and last, but not least, a species of symbiotic methane-generating bacteria. This last group of bacteria makes the Pelomyxa amoeba resemble a miniature cow in how it contains tiny methanogenic bacteria in its gut.

The Pelomyxa amoeba has no outward flagella or whip-like members that could propel it through the pond scum; it has tiny, non-functional undulipodia, or whip-like is inherited only through the mother, unlike DNA in the tails, near its edges instead. Since this amoeba doesn't have sex with other amoeba (i.e., doesn't exchange DNA), doesn't divide its nucleus by mitosis when it reproduces, and has no mitochondria[29], we can deduce from these facts that the invention of undulipodia, or whip-like tails, preceded the invention of all of these other features. All of the characteristics that Pelomyxa possesses puts this amoeba near the point where cancer originated on our Origin of Life timeline.

The methanogenic bacteria contained within the Pelomyxa exist in a symbiotic relationship with the giant amoeba; we believe that, in time, these methanogens and related bacteria, such as the methylotrophic (methane-oxidizing) bacteria, were absorbed into the very core of the cell itself and resulted in the cancer cell trait being a recessive trait in every living thing that evolved after Pelomyxa.[30]

SUMMARY

The process of endosymbiosis resulted in the cancer cell trait being incorporated into almost all life forms that evolved after the mycoplasma bacterium.

Endosymbiosis is the process of one bacterium engulfing another, then both deciding to live together in a mutually-beneficial relationship. (This is different from sex, which is the exchanging of DNA between two individuals.) We all owe a debt of gratitude to Pelomyxa[30] for surviving to the present day to provide us with much insight into how and when cancer originated.

Endosymbiosis is how mitochondria were formed. Interestingly, these tiny energy- generating organelles, or cell parts, have their own DNA that is separate from the DNA in the nucleus of the cell.

Endosymbiosis is how chloroplasts, the photosynthesizing parts of plant cells, were formed. These tiny bodies create carbohydrates from sunlight, carbon dioxide, and water and give off oxygen as a waste by-product. Without these organelles, all oxygen- breathing organisms would die.

One clue that cancer comes from a bacterium is how the E. coli bacteria produces toxins that kill cancer cells. This is because E.coli and the mycoplasma bacterium have been competitors or enemies for about three billion years.

Methanogenic bacteria are probably the main contributors to the endosymbiotic origins of the Cancer Cell trait. They are the first bacteria to use sterols to create internal membranes. Sterols are subsequently used by life forms to create their cell membranes, sex hormones, and other substances vital to life.

The Pelomyxa amoeba, which still exists today, illustrates how this endosymbiotic process worked a billion years ago or so. This amoeba contains methanogenic bacteria inside it surrounding its nuclei. These bacteria help the Pelomyxa digest its food, which consists mostly of one-celled bacteria, protists[31], and algae.

CHAPTER 7

THE CAUSES OF CANCER (REVISITED)

We will now examine the causes of cancer from a new perspective gained after our discussion on how cancer originated. Any theory on the origin of cancer must explain why such fundamentally dissimilar factors as chemicals, radiation, and viruses cause cancer. We think ours does, as you will soon see.

HOW CHEMICALS CAUSE CANCER

Nitrosamines

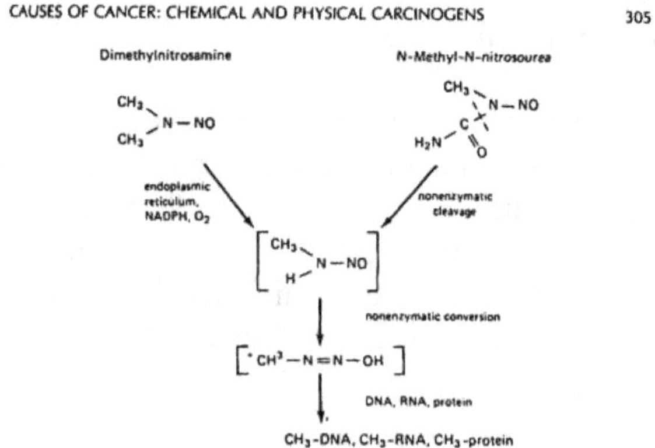

Figure 6-2 The enzymatic and nonenzymatic activations of dimethylnitrosamine and *N*-methyl-*N*-nitroso reactive nucleophiles.

"That inappropriate or unregulated demethylation of DNA can contribute to carcinogenesis is suggested by studies showing that chemical carcinogens or ultraviolet radiation can produce extensive demethylation, resulting in increased expression of quiescent genes in carcinogen-exposed cells."

[Source: *Cancer Biology* by Raymond Ruddon QZ200 R914c 1987 UCSD Biomedical Library]

The picture on the previous page shows how nitrosamine is converted through enzymatic and non-enzymatic action into a carcinogen. The carcinogen takes the form of a methane molecule bonding with DNA, RNA and protein molecules. Scientists now know how nitrosamine works to cause cancer (see the paragraph above, which is from Cancer Biology by Raymond Ruddon), but they don't know why it causes cancer. We believe that the reason why methane may play a part in carcinogenesis may be because the mycoplasma bacterium is an endosymbiotic descendant of the methane- producing Archaebacteria and the methane-eating Methylotrophic bacteria. This is why injecting the DNA of methanogenic bacteria into the nuclei of normal cells causes the cells to be transformed into cancer cells. [Source available upon request.] Methane was a much more important constituent of the atmosphere early in the evolution of the Earth. Here are the chemical constituents of Earth's atmosphere and oceans during that time period:

CH_4 (methane); NH_3 (ammonia); H_2O (water vapor); CO_2 (carbon dioxide); CO (carbon monoxide); NO (nitric oxide) – secondary atmosphere; NO_2 (nitrous oxide) – secondary atmosphere; SO_2 (sulfur dioxide) – secondary atmosphere; HCl (hydrochloric acid) – secondary atmosphere;

THE PRECURSOR TO CANCER CELLS

The list below shows the chemicals that methane-eating, or methane-oxidizing, bacteria either derive their energy from (List B), or create their cells and derive the energy they need from (List A). Presumably all of these chemicals were present in their environment when these bacteria evolved. Since most of these chemicals are carcinogens or promote carcinogenesis, we can deduce from this that the mycoplasma bacterium is related to these methane-oxidizing bacteria. Synthetic chemicals that are analogues of these chemicals are carcinogenic, too, because they can be converted by these bacteria into food or fuel after being broken down by enzymes or by other means.

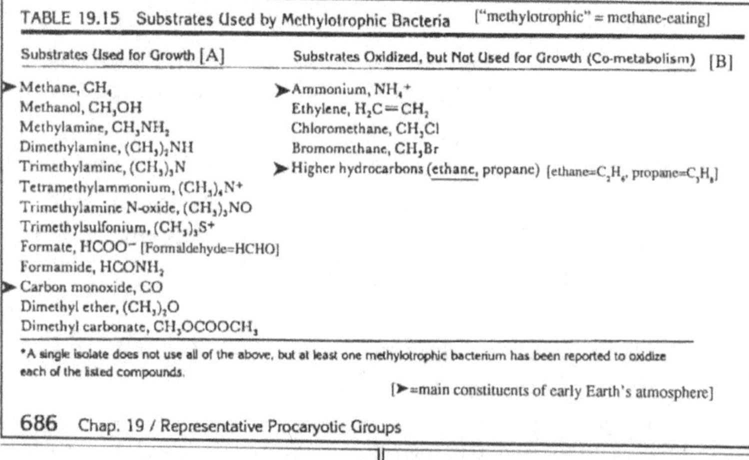

[From "Biology of Microorganisms, 4th Edition" by Thomas Brock, David Smith, and Michael Madigan 1984 Prentice-Hall QW4 B864B [BML]:]

TABLE 19.15 Substrates Used by Methylotrophic Bacteria ["methylotrophic" = methane-eating]

Substrates Used for Growth [A]	Substrates Oxidized, but Not Used for Growth (Co-metabolism) [B]
➤ Methane, CH_4	➤ Ammonium, NH_4^+
Methanol, CH_3OH	Ethylene, $H_2C{=}CH_2$
Methylamine, CH_3NH_2	Chloromethane, CH_3Cl
Dimethylamine, $(CH_3)_2NH$	Bromomethane, CH_3Br
Trimethylamine, $(CH_3)_3N$	➤ Higher hydrocarbons (<u>ethane</u>, propane) [ethane=C_2H_6, propane=C_3H_8]
Tetramethylammonium, $(CH_3)_4N^+$	
Trimethylamine N-oxide, $(CH_3)_3NO$	
Trimethylsulfonium, $(CH_3)_3S^+$	
Formate, $HCOO^-$ [Formaldehyde=HCHO]	
Formamide, $HCONH_2$	
➤ Carbon monoxide, CO	
Dimethyl ether, $(CH_3)_2O$	
Dimethyl carbonate, $CH_3OCOOCH_3$	

*A single isolate does not use all of the above, but at least one methylotrophic bacterium has been reported to oxidize each of the listed compounds.

[➤=main constituents of early Earth's atmosphere]

686   Chap. 19 / Representative Procaryotic Groups

Note that alcohol (methanol above and ethanol below) can be used by certain Methylobacteria for energy. This could explain why alcohol is a promoter of cancer, as the article below indicates:

From *Under the Influence,* by James Milam and
Katherine Ketcham. (1981). Bantam Books:

"The clinical association of long-term ingestion of large
amounts of alcoholic beverages (chronic alcoholism) with
a variety of cancers is known to most cancer
epidemiologists but is not widely recognized in the
medical profession.

"Alcohol is not a widely accepted cancer-causing agent,
but there are strong indications that large amounts of
alcohol taken over a prolonged period of time definitely
contribute to or aggravate cancers throughout the body.
Alcoholics appear to have an increased risk of head and
neck, esophageal, lung, and liver cancers. In each of these
cancers, alcohol probably acts in a different way,
sometimes directly affecting the cells, other times
indirectly increasing the cells' susceptibility to cancer.

There are a number of ways alcohol appears to contribute
to cancer:

By directly irritating the cells, thus targeting an area which
may then be more vulnerable to cancer.

By damaging the liver so that the ability to break down
and neutralize poisonous substances is greatly reduced.
The accumulation of these substances in the blood may
directly irritate the cells, increasing the likelihood of
cancer..."

HOW HORMONES AND CHOLESTEROL ARE INVOLVED IN CARCINOGENESIS

The reason why hormones such as estradiol, the most potent natural form of estrogen, and diethylstilbesterol (DES), a synthetic form of estrogen, may be carcinogenic in larger than normal doses could be because methane-oxidizing bacteria contain large amounts of sterols. From *The Biology of Microorganisms*, 4th Edition by Thomas Brock, David Smith, and Michael Madigan (1984) Prentice-Hall, we discover that:

"Most methane-oxidizing bacteria appear to be obligate methylotrophs, unable to utilize compounds with carbon-carbon bonds, but bacteria of one genus, Methylobacterium, are facultative methylotrophs, also being able to utilize organic acids, ethanol, and sugars [like our own cells].

"Methane-oxidizing bacteria are also unique among prokaryotes in possessing relatively large amounts of sterols. As we noted in Chapter 3, sterols are found in eukaryotes as a functional part of the membrane system, but seem to be absent from most prokaryotes. In the methane-oxidizing bacteria, sterols may be an essential part of the complete internal membrane system… that is involved in methane oxidation."

In other words, methane-oxidizing bacteria were the first bacteria with membranes (inner and outer) made of sterols. This places the methane-oxidizing bacteria on our timeline where the mycoplasma bacterium evolved.

The high sterol level in methane-oxidizing bacteria may explain why charred meat causes cancer. Charred meats contain high levels of oxidized cholesterol and are high in free radicals. When methane-oxidizing bacteria evolved, any cholesterol they contained would have been high in free radicals because it would have been bombarded with UV and other radiation from the sun, with the absence of an ozone layer in the Earth's atmosphere. Free radicals would have been much more abundant on the surface of the early Earth. (Please see the section on rancid fats in Chapter Two.) Human breast milk can be high in cholesterol epoxides, which may be a contributory factor in breast cancer, especially in Western women.

Studies in China examining the relationship between dietary intake and cancer incidence found that a high cholesterol diet increases the risk of cancer. Unfortunately, these studies did not examine whether the cholesterol was oxidized and whether breast cancer in Chinese women was related to the level of oxidized cholesterol in their breast milk. Recent articles1 seem to indicate that a Western-style diet changes the types of bacteria in breast tissue, which may have an effect on breast cancer rates.
Like most other bacteria, the mycoplasma bacterium evolved before nature invented sexual reproduction; that is, it reproduces asexually or by cloning instead. This is why we put the mycoplasma bacterium before "sexual reproduction begins" on the Origin of Life timeline in Chapter Four. This may explain why higher- than-normal sex hormone levels (both male and female hormone levels in both males and females) is a risk factor for cancer. The sex hormones are produced from cholesterol; if this

---

cholesterol is highly oxidized, it might increase the risk of sex hormone-related cancers such as breast, ovarian, and prostate cancer. Methanogenic bacteria is one of the few bacteria that uses cholesterol, according to this Wikipedia article. This is in line with our theory on the origin of cancer, which states that cancer is derived from the methanogenic bacteria, then it would make sense that cholesterol is involved in carcinogenesis. Around the time of the origin of cancer, nature invented skeletal structures and shells made from calcium carbonate. This is significant because microcalcification, or tiny calcium deposits in the breast, is how breast cancer is sometimes detected. This is another important clue that supports our theory and helps pinpoint when cancer entered the picture. Breast cancer cells are retrogressing to a previous stage when they first formed calcium carbonate-containing cell structures. This occurred around the time that nature invented the sex hormones and vitamin D, which are both made from cholesterol and which both work with calcium to form skeletons and shells.

HOW AND WHY RADIATION CAUSES CANCER

The picture at the top of the next page shows that all radiation from the sun below about 300 nanometers in wavelength is absorbed by the ozone layer. Back in Precambrian times there was no ozone layer, so much of this radiation fell unimpeded to the surface of the Earth. The mycoplasma bacterium, therefore, evolved under higher levels of UV, X-, and gamma-radiation, which is why we believe these forms of radiation cause cancer.

Why then is radiation used to treat cancer? At high enough doses, it will kill cancer cells. Interestingly, scientists have discovered that cancer cells that can survive in an environment of low oxygen can tolerate much higher doses of X-rays. (This is another clue that cancer cells evolve ved under both low-oxygen and high radiation conditions.)

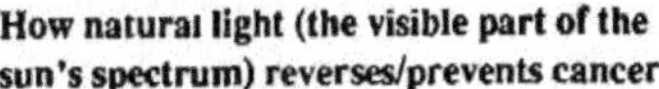

How natural light (the visible part of the sun's spectrum) reverses/prevents cancer:

[From "The Solar Wind and the Earth" edited by S. I. Akasofu & Y. Kamide 1987 Tera Scientific Publ. Co. QB529 .S627 [BML]:]

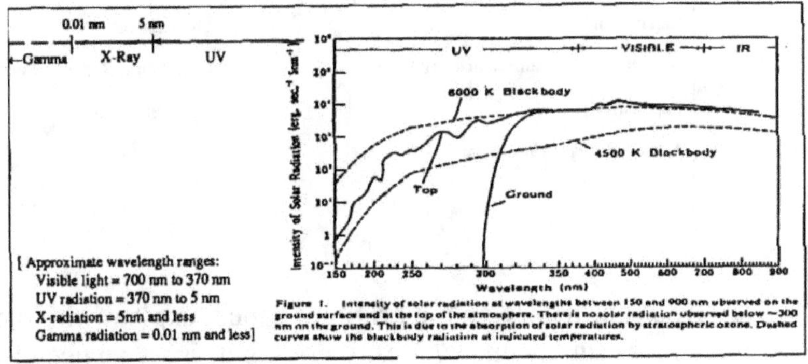

[Approximate wavelength ranges:
   Visible light = 700 nm to 370 nm
   UV radiation = 370 nm to 5 nm
   X-radiation = 5nm and less
   Gamma radiation = 0.01 nm and less]

Figure 1. Intensity of solar radiation at wavelengths between 150 and 900 nm observed on the ground surface and at the top of the atmosphere. There is no solar radiation observed below ~300 nm on the ground. This is due to the absorption of solar radiation by stratospheric ozone. Dashed curves show the blackbody radiation at indicated temperatures.

HOW AND WHY VIRUSES CAUSE CANCER

In Chapter Two, we briefly discussed the following viruses and the cancers they cause:

Virus	Type of Cancer
Epstein-Barr virus (also causes mononucleosis)	Pharyngeal cancer,
	Non-Hodgkin's Lymphoma
Helicobacter pylori* (also causes ulcers)	Stomach cancer
Hepatitis B	Liver cancer
HIV (Human Immunodeficiency Virus)	Lymphoma, Kaposi's Sarcoma
Papillomavirus	Cervical cancer
* actually, this is a bacterium	

Does our theory on the origin of cancer explain why these viruses cause cancer? Yes, it does, but, first, we need to explain what oncogenic retroviruses are and how they cause cancer.

ONCOGENIC RETROVIRUSES

Oncogenic retroviruses are a special class of cancer-causing viruses that work in a "retro" or backward fashion, i.e., instead of transmitting information from DNA to RNA, which is normally how things work in most cells, they use their RNA to modify the DNA of the cells they infect. They co-opt their host cell's DNA and cause it to create multiple copies of themselves. These copies then infect other cells in the body or other nearby organisms.

There are many different kinds of oncogenic retroviruses that infect a wide variety of plant and animal species. A partial list of these viruses is given below. Scientists have examined the RNA sequences of oncogenic retroviruses and have developed an evolutionary tree for these viruses:

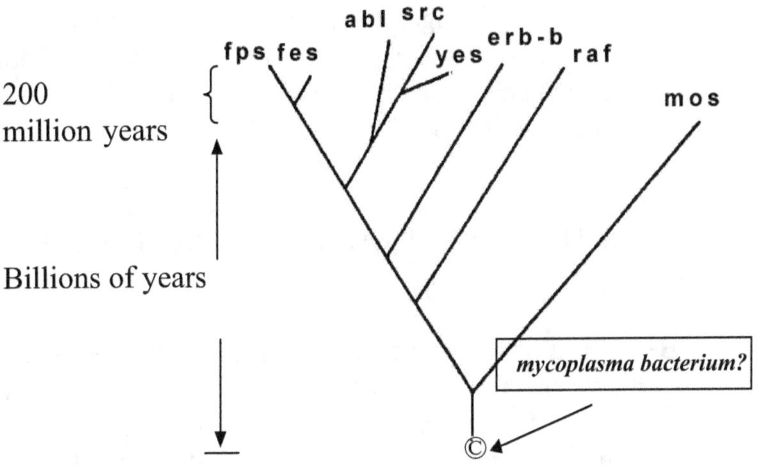

The book, *Cancer Biology* by Raymond Ruddon (1987), Oxford University Press, tells us that "These are very old genes, indeed, fps and fes, for example, appear to have diverged about 200 million years ago." We can deduce from this diagram that many oncogenic retroviruses probably share a common ancestor that existed billions of years ago. We think that common ancestor is the mycoplasma bacterium.

Viruses are believed to have originated from bacteria that have retrogressed and given up parts of the cell that are necessary for metabolism, because all they really need is their DNA or RNA and very little else. They are capable of entering a dormant stage by creating spores; these spores resemble crystals and seem to be a transitional form between life and non-life. They seem to point to a possible inorganic origin for life. We think it is very likely that the mycoplasma bacterium retrogressed into the common ancestor of all oncogenic retroviruses. Viruses that cause diseases other than cancer are probably the result of non-mycoplasma bacteria retrogressing and giving up cell parts that they don't need.

A PARTIAL LIST OF ONCOGENIC RETROVIRUSES

Below is a list of common retroviruses with those that are found in the evolutionary tree above marked with arrows in the far left column. The oncogenes that these retroviruses contain exist in the DNA of nearly all living things on Earth and go back billions of years to a common ancestor that we all share: the mycoplasma bacterium.

Table 7-2 Viral oncogenes contained in the genomes of oncogenic retroviruses[a]

Oncogene	Virus	Species of origin
→ *abl*	Abelson murine leukemia virus	Mouse
→ *fes*[b]	ST feline sarcoma virus	Cat
→ *fps*[b]	Fujinami sarcoma virus	Chicken
fgr	Gardner–Rasheed feline sarcoma virus	Cat
ros	UR II avian sarcoma virus	Chicken
→ *src*	Rous sarcoma virus	Chicken
→ *yes*	Y73 sarcoma virus	Chicken
→ *erb-B*	Avian erythroblastosis virus	Chicken
fms	McDonough feline sarcoma virus	Cat
→ *raf*[b]	3611 Murine sarcoma virus	Mouse
mil(mht)[b]	MH2 virus	Chicken
→ *mos*	Moloney murine sarcoma virus	Mouse
sis	Simian sarcoma virus	Woolly monkey
Ha-ras	Harvey murine sarcoma virus	Rat
Ki-ras	Kirsten murine sarcoma virus	Rat
fos	FBJ osteosarcoma virus	Mouse
myb	Avian myeloblastosis virus	Chicken
myc	MC29 myelocytomatosis virus	Chicken
erb-A	Avian erythroblastosis virus	Chicken
ets	E26 virus	Chicken
rel	Reticuloendotheliosis virus	Turkey
ski	Avian SKV770 virus	Chicken

[a]The names of the viral oncogenes are loosely derived from the names of the viruses in which they were identified or from the types of cancers they cause (*src* from Rous sarcoma virus or *ras* from rat sarcoma, for example). A half-dozen or so additional transforming genes, some related to the viral oncogenes and some not, have been identified. In addition, the early region genes E1A and E1B of adenoviruses, as well as the T antigens of SV 40 and polyoma viruses, are considered oncogenes.

[b]*fes* and *fps* are feline and avian versions of the same oncogene; *raf* and *mil(mht)* are murine and avian oncogene counterparts.

(Modified from Marx.[17])

So there is a common thread that links all three major factors that cause cancer, and that common thread is the mycoplasma bacterium.

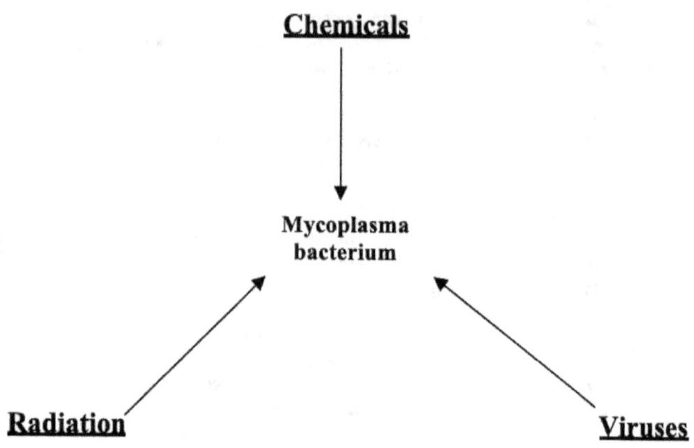

This is a more meaningful diagram:

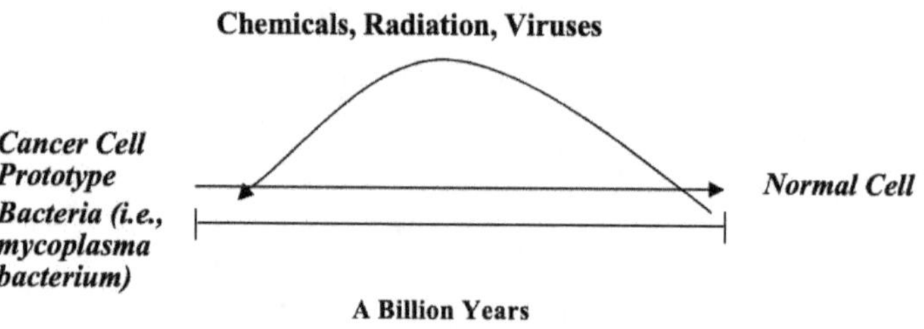

SUMMARY

Our theory on the origin of cancer explains why such seemingly unrelated factors such as chemicals, radiation, and viruses cause cancer. The reason why they cause cancer is because they cause normal cells to revert back to the mycoplasma bacterium way of life.

This is why demethylation can contribute to carcinogenesis; cells that turn cancerous are manifesting their methanogenic or methane-eating bacterial heritage.

The reason why hormones cause cancer may be because methanogenic bacteria are high in sterols, and hormones are made from cholesterol. Note that the mycoplasma bacterium evolved before nature invented sexual reproduction, when life was still reproducing asexually (i.e., by cloning).

The reason why viruses cause cancer is because viruses are stripped-down bacteria that have lost body (cell) parts that they don't need. The class of viruses that cause cancer, which are called oncogenic retroviruses, could be descendants of a stripped-down mycoplasma bacterium. Radiation causes cancer because the mycoplasma bacterium evolved when there was very little oxygen in the atmosphere, and there was no ozone layer. It evolved under high UV-, gamma-, and cosmic-radiation conditions.

CHAPTER 8

THE PREVENTION OF CANCER (REVISITED)

We will now examine the factors that prevent cancer mentioned in Chapter Three from a new perspective gained from our theory on the origin of cancer.

FREE RADICALS

To recapitulate what we learned about free radicals in Chapter Three, oxygen free radicals are oxygen molecules that are deficient in electrons. They are generated as a by-product of oxygen-based metabolism and by UV-radiation hitting oxygen atoms. Ideally, oxygen and other molecules like to keep their electrons in pairs. Free radicals create electron pairs by stealing electrons from other molecules, damaging them in the process.

Antioxidants work by giving up their electrons to stabilize free radicals and prevent them from damaging DNA and other parts of the cell. The most effective antioxidants are vitamins, provitamins (or precursors to vitamin A, such as betacarotene), elements such as selenium and zinc, and enzymes such as superoxide dismutase and glutathione. How do vitamins work to prevent free radicals? What are vitamins? Where do they come from?

VITAMINS

Vitamins are chemical substances usually required in extremely small doses to facilitate chemical reactions involved in metabolism and other bodily functions. These substances must generally be obtained from outside the body; they usually cannot be made by the body (a notable exception being vitamin D, which is made in our skin from sunlight and cholesterol). Vitamins are used to process carbohydrates, proteins, and fats. Conveniently, they are usually found in the foods where they are needed. Together with minerals, they are absolutely essential to health.

Where do vitamins come from? Our theory on the origin of cancer provides the answer to this question. Back in the Precambrian era when life was originating on Earth, there would have been an abundance of free radicals with the ozone layer not yet fully formed and photosynthetic organisms like cyanobacteria beginning to grow in numbers, spewing forth more and more free oxygen into the atmosphere. Nature had to invent substances to prevent free radicals and the oxidizing atmosphere from damaging cell parts. These substances were vitamins and other antioxidants like superoxide dismutase. The cell parts that were fatty or oily required fat-soluble vitamins like vitamins A, D, E, and K; the cell parts that were water-based required water-soluble vitamins like vitamins B and C.

Vitamin D is a good example of an antioxidant naturally produced in the skin (a fatty part of the body) by sunlight. It is a protective vitamin that also works with calcium and phosphorus to form our skeletons and teeth. Vitamin E is another important oil-based antioxidant that prevents the

spoiling or oxidation of oil- or fat-based substances in our
bodies.

DRUGS

Taxol, Tamoxifen (cholesterol-lowering drug)

How could something that comes from the bark of a yew
tree work against cancer? The reason why Taxol prevents
cancer or causes a regression in cancer is because this
chemical substance acts like an anti-estrogen. Recall that
estrogen is formed from cholesterol. Both plants and
animals use sterols to form membranes; the bark of a tree
is another type of membrane. The function of the bark is to
protect the internal contents of the tree from the
environment, just as the membrane of a cell protects the
internal contents of the cell from its micro-environment.
Lipoproteins (cholesterol) are ideal molecules for a
membrane because they can handle both water-based and
oil-based molecules, allowing their passage through the
membrane as needed.

Cis-platinum (Cisplatin), catalytic converters

Cisplatin binds to parts of DNA and interferes with the
dividing of cells. There are mechanisms in the body to
detect faulty cells that cause these cells to commit suicide.
Cisplatin is especially effective in the treatment of
testicular cancer. Another possible factor that helps
Cisplatin fight cancer is that it may increase the uptake of

oxygen by cells (recall that cancer cells can exist happily in low-oxygen environments), just like they do in catalytic converters in automobiles to reduce noxious emissions.

Methotrexate

Methotrexate belongs to a group of drugs known as antimetabolites and is used to treat cancers of the breast, head and neck, lung, blood, bone, lymph, and uterus. This drug works by blocking the action of an enzyme known as dihydrofolate reductase in cancer cells. Methotrexate may be related to chemicals produced by bacteria that are competitors of the mycoplasma bacterium.

5-fluorouracil, etc.

The family of drugs represented by 5-fluorouracil works by interfering with the process of meiosis or DNA division in the cell. 5-fluorouracil may also be related to noxious chemicals produced by bacteria that are competitors of the mycoplasma bacterium.

RADIATION

Natural (visible) light; UV, and Ionizing radiation (Gamma, X-ray, and Cosmic)

Ultraviolet and ionizing radiation can interact with DNA and cause normal cells to turn cancerous. In one experiment with the fish Poecilia formosa, cancerous cells can be induced to become normal cells again by exposure to visible light. Because cancer cells evolved under high UV-radiation conditions, we would expect that UV radiation would induce this cancerous reversion process.

When some cancerous cells are exposed to normal, visible (full-spectrum) light, they revert to being normal cells again. This is also what we would expect from our theory on the origin of cancer (and it gives us hope that exposure to natural light may be an important adjunctive treatment for cancer patients).

Heat, hyperthermia, thermophilic bacteria

At one time, scientists were hopeful that raising the temperature of cancer patients would help reduce the size of their tumors. This form of treatment has largely been abandoned now, but there may be some validity to it. It is possible that, for some cancers, hyperthermia may work. The reason why it may work could be because cancer cells are derived from a line of bacteria that competed with thermophilic bacteria. (They are not in a direct line of succession from that group of bacteria.) It is possible that they favor a cooler micro-environment.

Exercise

The reason why exercise may help prevent cancer is because it has the following effects:

Exercise increases the uptake of oxygen by the cells of the body. Cancer cells don't grow, or their growth slows, when they are exposed to higher levels of oxygen.

Exercise decreases the production of sex hormones. As we saw earlier, the sex hormones promote the growth of some cancer cells.

Exercise decreases the levels of circulating cholesterol, and especially the bad form of cholesterol, or the LDL cholesterol. (This is related to #2, because the sex hormones are produced from cholesterol.)

Exercise improves the effectiveness of insulin and lowers the levels of blood sugar. Consumed sugar increases the production of estrogen in the stomach by certain bacteria.

Chlorophyll

This green coloring matter in plants and leaves is essential to the production of carbohydrates by photosynthesis. Chlorophyll absorbs the energy of UV and ionizing radiation that creates free radicals. It also produces oxygen as a waste by-product of the carbohydrate-production process, so it has a "double-whammy" effect against cancer. Chlorophyll is another one of those inventions that nature devised to absorb the harmful rays of the sun before the ozone layer formed.

Indoles, illudin (mushrooms), diallyl disulphide (garlic)

Broccoli and other cruciferous vegetables contain a substance called sulforaphane, which kills the Helicobacter pylori bacterium. This bacterium causes stomach ulcers, which can eventually result in stomach cancer. Cruciferous vegetables also contain indoles, which can transform carcinogens into harmless substances. The reason why a sulfur-based substance like sulforaphane could work against the Helicobacter bacterium is because this bacterium is probably a descendant of the mycoplasma bacterium and is not in the direct line of succession of the sulfate bacteria group. (Please see the Evolutionary Tree diagram in Chapter Six.)

Lactobacilli (miso soup, yogurt), Tuberculosis bacillus, E. Coli

Lactobacilli, the tuberculosis bacillus, and E. Coli have anti-cancer properties because all of these bacteria are competitors to the mycoplasma bacterium. In other words, these bacteria compete with the methanogenic line of bacteria from which the mycoplasma bacterium is derived. This is why they produce substances that attack and kill cancer cells.

Phytoestrogens (plant estrogens)

Soy beans contain phytoestrogens that replace the body's own estrogens, protecting against breast and ovarian cancers. Soy beans also contain genistein, which can block the supply of blood to tumors. In an article appearing in the March 4, 1998 issue of the Journal of the National Cancer Institute, Amy Lee, professor of biochemistry and molecular biology and the associate director of basic research at the USC/Norris Comprehensive Cancer Center, explains how genistein turns off the defense mechanism that cells use when they are stressed, such as by oxygen-deprivation, starvation, malnutrition, infection, and extreme heat. Cells turn on stress response genes to protect the body under these conditions.[32] Our theory on the origin of cancer would explain these stress response genes as genes that are descended from those that are found in the mycoplasma bacterium. The stress response genes turn on when the micro-environment reminds the cell of its mycoplasma bacterium days.

SUMMARY

The formation of free radicals is prevented by vitamins, minerals such as selenium, and enzymes, such as superoxide dismutase.

Vitamins are chemical substances required in micro-doses in most cases which help in the chemical reactions that make life possible.

Nature had to invent vitamins and other anti-oxidants to counteract increasing levels of oxygen in the atmosphere after the birth of the photosynthetic organisms, such as the cyanobacteria.

Many of the drugs (such as methotrexate and cisplatin) and other factors we use (such as lactobacillus) to fight cancer are effective because they contain or produce analogues of substances produced by bacterial competitors of the mycoplasma bacterium.

UV radiation, cosmic radiation, and X-rays cause normal cells to turn cancerous because they remind the cells of their mycoplasma bacterium origins. The mycoplasma bacterium evolved when there were higher levels of these forms of radiation, because there was not yet an ozone layer.

The reason why phytoestrogens, sex hormones, and cholesterol play a part in carcinogenesis is because the mycoplasma bacterium is a direct descendant of the methanogenic bacteria, which are high in sterols. Their internal membranes are made of sterols; in fact, they were the first bacteria to use sterols for membranes. Our cell membranes are made from cholesterol, too. The sex hormones are made from sterols, as is our skin. The skin contains about 11% by weight of the cholesterol in our bodies.

CHAPTER 9

THE FUTURE FOR CANCER

Why does cancer exist? We believe that cancer exists because the conditions that were present for the formation of life on this planet and for the origin of cancer, which were very different from those that exist today, may someday return. There may be a survival advantage for living cells to retain the mycoplasma bacterium way of life. There is no survival advantage, of course, for the organism in which the cancer exists, and this is why there are mechanisms in place in most higher organisms to destroy cells that turn cancerous, as we saw with lymphocytes in Chapter One.

It is ironic that cancer usually occurs in older people, because cells that turn cancerous are returning to the way they were when they were young, in fact, to when cells first evolved. This makes sense because these cells are trying to survive when conditions around them are less than ideal–when the oxygen level in their microenvironment is reduced, when fewer nutrients exist, and when they are being attacked by free radicals–by reverting to a way of life that allowed them to survive under these same conditions eons ago.

What occurs in older people with cancer, unfortunately, is occurring on a global scale right now. As more and more species go extinct, primarily from the loss of habitat, introduced non-native species, over-fishing/over-harvesting, and the introduction of genetically-modified organisms, there could be a massive die-off or "extinction event" of key species, such as some bacteria, plankton or bees, which pollinate many plant species. The whole intricate, complex house of cards that supports life on this planet could collapse, leaving only extremely hardy and adaptable species like certain microorganisms. Conditions would then more closely resemble those that existed on the early Earth, as oxygen levels decrease and carbon dioxide (and methane) levels increase. The ozone layer would be greatly reduced and UV levels would increase at the surface of the Earth, just as they did during the formative stages of the planet Earth. The Earth may then more closely resemble Venus and Mars, where the atmosphere is over 90% carbon dioxide.[33] For these and other reasons, there may be a survival advantage for life to retain the ability to return to the mycoplasma bacterium way of life.

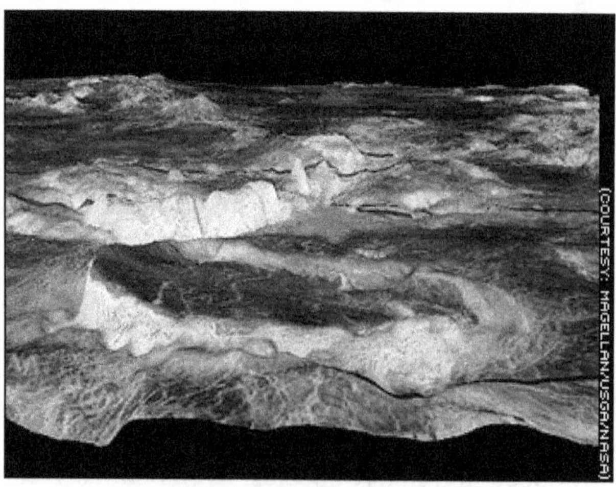

Photo: The surface of Venus (taken with radar by a satellite orbiting the planet)

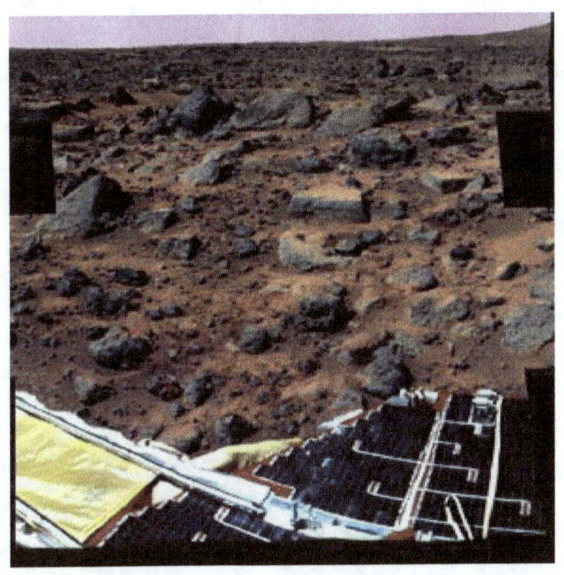

Photo: A view from the Mars Pathfinder Lander of the
landscape of Mars at the Sagan Memorial Station
(an enhanced color image).

SUMMARY

Ironically, cancer exists because the conditions that
favored the origin of life (conditions that are toxic to most
present-day life) favor the Cancer Cell way of life. Cancer
is part and parcel of the process of life originating on this
planet.

These conditions may yet return to the Earth, so there is a
survival advantage for cells to retain the Cancer Cell way
of life. These conditions include a lowering of the oxygen
level, an increase in the CO_2 level, an increase in free
radicals—in short, conditions that are similar to those that
exist on other planets like Mars, Venus, and Europa.

Mars may, in fact, be how the Earth will look like in a billion years (or sooner, if we aren't careful).

CHAPTER 10

THE BEST CANCER PREVENTION STRATEGY

CONFUSION REIGNS

It is hard to know sometimes exactly what we should and shouldn't be eating, because there is so much shifting and constantly changing information in the media and elsewhere. We think the best strategy to follow in preventing cancer is to see how the information fits our theory on the origin of cancer and how it fits in with our biological and evolutionary heritage. This means that we should learn how our distant and more recent ancestors ate and lived, how healthy they were, and what sort of diseases they had. We've done exactly that, and this is what we've learned:

Milk - Our Paleolithic ancestors consumed very little milk or dairy products, and yet they had very little osteoporosis. In fact, the gene to digest lactose, the sugar in milk, is a fairly recent development in humans. This gene evolved only about 8,000 years ago in humans living in the northern Mesopotamian region in present-day Iraq. Most Asians, blacks, and some Mediterranean peoples cannot digest milk because they lack this gene.

Meat - Our ancestors ate very little meat. We believe, however, that it is unrealistic to expect people to give up beef and other meat, and probably unnecessary. If the quantities are kept small or the cuts lean, it is probably healthy to consume some red meat. However, the Atkins Diet and similar diets, in which carbohydrates are severely restricted and protein intake is increased, is probably not a good idea, because it lacks fiber and increases the cholesterol level (and especially the oxidized forms of cholesterol) and may give people the mistaken impression that meats and fats are the only foods we need.

Wheat - Our ancestors ate very little wheat and virtually no processed foods made from wheat, such as bread and pasta. It has only been within the last 10,000 years or so that humans have become a settled, agrarian species. Before that, we were hunter- gatherers who moved from place to place living off the land. Why then do we seem to crave foods like bread, pasta, corn, and rice? The short answer is that they are simple carbohydrates that are easily digested and that quickly raise our blood sugar levels. Our bodies only have a four- to six-hour store of carbohydrates, mostly in the liver, so most people feel compelled to replenish their store of carbohydrates after that amount of time.

Is it true that hunter-gatherers suffer less from chronic, degenerative diseases like cancer and heart disease? Some scientists who have studied present-day hunter-gatherers in the world have determined this to be the case. A good example of this is the Bushmen of the Kalahari in Africa. The Bushmen are a nomadic tribe of Paleolithic-age hunter- gatherers. Their favorite foods, such as the mongongo nut, are high in protein, B- vitamins, fiber, flavonoids, and antioxidants, and low in fat with little or no cholesterol.

Exercise - There have been many studies showing that one of the best ways to prevent cancer (such as breast cancer) is through exercise. Our Paleolithic ancestors led physically demanding lives; they were hunter-gatherers who were always on the move, seeking out fresh hunting and gathering grounds. Their bodies craved fat and sweets, just as ours do, but they never got fat, because they had much higher energy expenditures than we do, and ate foods with very little fat and sugar.

The Okinawa Program - from *The Okinawa Program* by Bradley J. Wilcox, M.D.; D. Craig Wilcox, Ph.D.; and Makoto Suzuki, M.D. (2001) Three Rivers Press/Random House. Senior citizens who live on Okinawa still practice their traditional diets and now have the longest average lifespan in the world. (The Japanese have the second longest average lifespans.) Prostate cancer and breast cancer are almost unheard of. Their longevity and good health are not solely due to their diets, of course, but here are the basic features of their diet:

- Very high in sweet potato (*imo, numu* in Japanese).

- Extremely high in soy foods containing flavonoids (an antioxidant), such as tofu and miso soup.
- Very few dairy products (very little butter, very little cheese).

- Very little meat, mainly pork and poultry.

- High in fish (extremely fresh, just caught).

- High in vegetables (approximately 80% of their diet is plant-based).

- Some fruits, such as watermelon, Asian pears, and cantaloupe.

- The use of monounsaturated fats, mostly canola oil, which is high in Omega-3 oils (as is fish). Very little fried foods, mostly stir-fried with canola oil.

- Seaweeds (high in betacarotene, fiber, calcium, and iron), turmeric, and other herbs and spices.
- They believe in the practice of leaving the table with less than a full stomach.

- Very little refined, processed foods, except for white rice.

What if you aren't Asian? Will the "Okinawa Program" work for you? We think that it will, but you and your body are the best judge of which foods work best for you (for example, some people are allergic to soy products). You should consult a nutritionist or physician who is knowledgeable about nutrition for the best advice. We believe that the general principles outlined in the "Okinawa Program" are what is most important.

THE BEST WAYS TO PREVENT CANCER

What then are the best ways overall to prevent cancer? Here are some practical steps that we can all take:

DIET

Everything you eat should be as fresh as possible. Spoiled, moldy, or rancid foods, especially if they contain rancid fats or oils, are high in carcinogens. Throw out perishables that are more than three days old or put them on the compost pile unless they are meat, bones, or foods high in grease or oil. Reduce your consumption of preserved foods unless they are fermented. (See #6 below.) Choose fresh, raw foods over canned or even frozen foods. Just picked is even better. (We recommend growing your own vegetables and fruits, if possible.)

Reduce your consumption of deep-fat fried foods, especially French fries, which are often made in old, rancid oil. Reduce your consumption of beef and pork, which are high in fat, much of which is polyunsaturated and becomes rancid more quickly. Eat more fresh fish, lamb, fowl, and wild game.

Increase your consumption of foods high in vitamin C: oranges, limes, lemons, green peppers, ripe tomatoes, etc. Use natural vitamin C powder mixed into freshly-squeezed orange juice to increase your vitamin C intake. Also, add some lemon juice from fresh lemons into the orange juice to provide a more complete intake of vitamin C and the synergistically-acting bioflavonoids (sometimes called vitamin P). Vitamin C is vital in keeping the immune system functioning properly.

Avoid fat and sugar. Avoid margarine completely; it is high in polyunsaturated, hydrogenated fat (a totally artificial form of fat) and usually has artificial coloring and flavoring. Butter or olive oil, used sparingly, is better. Reduce your intake of processed oils, mayonnaise, salad dressings, etc.

Reduce your consumption of salt (except in miso soup, see #6 below), because cancerous cells are high in sodium, low in potassium, which is the exact opposite of normal cells. Vegetables, fruits, and cereals are high in potassium. Eat organic produce that is unsprayed with pesticides so that you don't have to wash them very much; potassium is water soluble and is easily lost by soaking or washing the fruits and vegetables in water. Avoid water softeners that add sodium and remove vital minerals such as calcium and magnesium in the water. Drink hard water that contains these minerals; use bottled spring water, if local water is soft or polluted.

Eat more fermented foods, especially miso soup and low-fat yogurt without sugar, fructose, honey, etc. These foods contain lactobacillus and other bacteria which have antitumor and cholesterol-reducing properties.

Increase your consumption of yellow, orange, and dark green vegetables and fruits, which are high in beta-carotene (pre-vitamin A), a potent anticarcinogen, such as:

Butternut squash, golden acorn squash, spaghetti squash, and other squashes,
Cantaloupe, papaya, mango, and other tropical fruits,
Carrots, parsnips, and related vegetables,
Peaches, apricots, plums, and nectarines,

Seaweeds, as in sushi-nori, kombu, hijiki, wakame, in Japanese, Spinach, beet greens, dandelion greens, amaranth greens, turnip greens,
collard greens, swiss chard and kale, Sweet potatoes, yams, and other potatoes.

Increase your consumption of chlorophyll and folic acid, i.e., green vegetables: alfalfa sprouts, other sprouts, lettuce (dark green kinds), spinach, Swiss chard, kale, collard greens, cabbage, broccoli, and peas. Chlorophyll has free radical-reducing properties. Free radicals are extremely reactive molecules thought to cause mutations in DNA resulting in cancer. Folic acid, one of the B-vitamins, is necessary for many of the metabolic processes in the body, including the synthesis of DNA and RNA; thus, folic acid is vital for proper cell growth and division. Folic acid deficiency is one of the most common vitamin deficiencies and may be partly responsible for the high rates of cancer in this country.

Increase your fiber intake: oat bran or oatmeal, rice bran or brown rice, wheat bran or whole wheat products, beans, lentils, cucumbers, broccoli, barley, and other grains unless you have digestive problems with gluten. Other foods that are high in fiber include dried apricots, prunes, figs, kumquats and artichokes. Fiber reduces stool transit time by providing bulk, which helps speed up the elimination of carcinogens from the intestinal tract. Fiber may therefore help prevent colon cancer. Fiber also reduces blood cholesterol levels.

Increase your intake of cruciferous vegetables: broccoli, cauliflower, cabbage, and brussel sprouts. These vegetables contain chemicals that have antitumor properties. They also provide calcium from a non-dairy source, which will help prevent certain forms of cancer, such as colon cancer.

Increase your consumption of tomatoes and tomato sauce. Tomatoes contain lycopene, which is a potent antioxidant that appears to protect against prostate cancer.

Try to eat more soy beans and soy bean products, such as tofu and miso, unless you are allergic to soy products. Soy beans contain genistein, which protects against breast cancer by binding to estrogen receptor sites and blocking the activity of estrogen.

Try green tea instead of soft drinks. (Green tea does have caffeine, so it may not be for everyone. Many soft drinks have caffeine, too.) Green tea contains polyphenols, which are potent antioxidants. It also contain catechins, which inhibit the growth of new blood vessels, thus impeding the flow of nutrients to tumors.

Increase your consumption of blueberries and other berries. They contain anthocyanins that prevent free radical damage linked to heart disease and cancer.

Eat more avocado, which is one of the richest sources of the antioxidant glutathione, which helps reduce free radicals and blocks the absorption of harmful fats in the intestinal tract.

Eat more garlic, onions, chives and asparagus. These foods contain selenium, which has anti-cancer properties. (Other sources of selenium include seafood and meats.) They also contain diallyl disulphides, which are believed to prevent cancer.

Consume more nuts unless you are allergic to certain nuts. Nuts, such as pecans and walnuts, contain a chemical called ellagic acid. In studies, ellagic acid causes apoptosis, where cells that turn cancerous or that have mutations commit suicide. Nuts also reduce the levels of the bad LDL cholesterol and increase the levels of the good HDL cholesterol. In addition, they are high in the antioxidant vitamin E.

Eat more seafood, such as salmon, herring, mackerel, and bluefish. These fish contain high levels of omega-3 fish oils, because of their position at the top of a marine food chain beginning with algae that are high in omega-3 fatty acids. Omega-3 fatty acids lower the levels of triglycerides and the bad form of cholesterol (LDL) in the blood and seem to reduce inflammation, which may be a factor in heart disease and cancer, as well as in autoimmune diseases, such as arthritis.

Reduce your alcohol consumption if you drink. Alcohol may be a promoter of cancer by altering hormone levels in the body. Some cancers, such as breast and prostate cancer, are related to elevated levels of certain hormones in the body.

Reduce your caloric intake. Reduce your body weight if you are overweight. Studies on laboratory animals show that caloric restriction extends their life spans significantly and reduces the incidence of tumors. Also, breast cancer mortality rates seem to be directly proportional to fat and sugar intake, and also to body mass (height and weight). So eat small portions of highly nutritious, but low in fat foods that are as fresh and unprocessed as possible.

EXERCISE

Increase your energy expenditure. Exercise improves elimination of toxins, blood circulation, and oxygen intake (uptake)–all of which are believed to be beneficial in warding off cancer. Also, exercise, along with caloric restriction, is the fastest and best way to lose weight. If you find it hard to motivate yourself to exercise, find a friend or relative to join you.

Avoid excessive stress. Stress increases cortisol levels in the body which boosts blood sugar levels and suppresses the immune system. Stress alone can often bring on disease. Exercise reduces stress through the production of endorphins, which are natural opiate- like substances, in the brain, but both exercise and stress "burn up" the B-vitamins, so be sure to increase your intake of the B-complex vitamins.

OXYGEN INTAKE

As mentioned above, exercise increases oxygen levels in the body, but does this more effectively if you exercise outdoors.

Sleep in a well-aerated room for maximum oxygen uptake during our body's rest and repair period. Although rarely possible for most people, sleeping outdoors in a secure, enclosed porch, room, cabaña, or tent would be even better. Studies show that cancerous cells don't grow, or their growth slows, if they are bathed in high levels of oxygen.

Avoid as much pollution as possible, including pollution found in the home, office, or elsewhere from carcinogenic chemicals used in the workplace or from harmful chemicals (such as formaldehyde) "outgassing" from plastic or pressboard furniture, building materials, copying or blueprint machines, paint, smokers, and so on. The liberal use of houseplants inside your home and office will help to clear the air of toxins.

NATURAL LIGHT

Increase your exposure to natural light, but don't overdo it, especially if you are light- skinned. Cancerous cells don't grow, or their growth slows, when they are exposed to visible light. Also, our eyes contain receptors that stimulate the production of certain hormones–including our sex hormones–but only if these receptors are exposed to natural light, which is usually much more intense and has a different spectral characteristic than artificial lighting. Altered hormone levels in the body could be responsible for some forms of cancer. Avoid long exposure to undiffused fluorescent light, which may cause skin cancer. Spend more time outdoors. On hot, sunny days, stay more in the shade to avoid sunstroke, sunburn and possible skin cancer later.

Exposure to natural light has been found to suppress appetite and weight gain.

Sleep in a completely dark room for maximum production of hormones, such as melatonin, needed for the deepest, most restful sleep. (Melatonin also happens to be a powerful antioxidant.) Sleep disturbances could be responsible for weight gain and other health problems.

SUMMARY

The bottom line on preventing cancer seems to be reducing the intake of animal products and processed or manufactured foods and increasing the consumption of plant products, especially colorful fruits and vegetables and soy products, such as tofu, miso, and edamame, which are boiled green soy beans.

Other possible preventive factors are the consumption of seafood/EPA (eicosapentaenoic acid), and mono-unsaturated oils, such as olive oil and avocados. Avoiding trans-fatty acids, hydrogenated fats in margarines and processed foods, and oxidized (burnt) cholesterol and fats may also be useful.

Eating more fermented foods such as miso, sauerkraut, and yogurt may help prevent cancer. These lactobacilli-containing foods seem to have potent anti-cancer properties.

Consuming anti-estrogens like soy products, unless you are allergic to soy, may help prevent breast cancer.

Reducing total caloric consumption may help prevent cancers of all types. Pushing away from the dinner table before you are completely full may be a good policy to follow.

Exercise seems to prevent cancer, especially the hormone-related cancers such as breast cancer and prostate cancer.

Stress-reduction is another preventative factor that may help.

Maintaining a social network seems to be important, not only to our overall health, but to preventing cancer.

TABLE OF ENDNOTES

[1] *Cancer Facts & Figures 2020.* American Cancer Society.

[2] dead, black

[3] which could mean that close to 100% of the population has cancer

[4] in the laboratory. Some bacteria show this same characteristic; they can become tolerant to certain antibiotics and drugs used to control them.

[5] Although this has been disputed

[6] Fermentation = the anaerobic enzymatic conversion of organic compounds, especially carbohydrates, to simpler compounds, especially to ethyl alcohol, resulting in energy in the form of adenosine triphosphate(ATP); the process is used in the production of alcohol, bread, and vinegar, and other food or industrial products…Fermentation occurs widely in bacteria and yeasts…

[7] Glycolysis = the anaerobic enzymatic conversion of glucose to the simpler compounds lactate or pyruvate, resulting in energy stored in the form of adenosine triphosphate (ATP), as occurs in muscle; it differs from respiration in that organic substances, rather than molecular oxygen, are used as electron acceptors (Source: *Dorland's Illustrated Medical Dictionary, 27th Edition*)

[8] see the section below for an explanation of what endosymbiosis is

[9] facultative aerobic = can live with or without oxygen

[10] A beta particle = a high speed electron or positron, especially one emitted in radioactive decay

[11] [Blank]

[12] Muramic acid = the characteristic starch or cellulose composing bacterial cell walls

[13] *Endo* means "within" and *symbiosis* means "any mutually beneficial relationship between two organisms, persons, groups, etc.

[14] The dictionary definition of mitochondria is a spherical or elongated organelle in the cytoplasm of nearly all eukaryotic cells, containing genetic material and many enzymes important for cell metabolism, including those responsible for the conversion of food to usable energy.

[15] Protista are animal-like and plant-like unicellular organisms with distinct nuclei, i.e., the eukaryotes, including protozoa, algae (except the blue-green algae or bacteria), and certain intermediate forms. In some classification systems, protista includes only the protozoa.

[16] Tobacco plants, for example, can contract "Crown Gall" disease

[17] bacteria with a distinct nucleus

[18] Nucleotides = any of a group of molecules that, when linked together, form the building blocks of DNA or RNA, composed of a phosphate group, the bases adenine, cytosine, guanosine, and thymine, and a pentose sugar, in RNA, the thymine base being replaced by uracil

[19] Gene = the basic physical unit of heredity; a linear sequence of nucleotides along a segment of DNA that provides the coded instructions for synthesis of RNA, which, when translated into protein, leads to the expression of hereditary character. [Source: *The Random House Dictionary of the English Language, Second Edition Unabridged* 1987.]

[20] The Rosetta Stone = a basalt tablet bearing inscriptions in Greek and in Egyptian hieroglyphics that was discovered in 1799 near Rosetta, a northern Egyptian town located in the Nile River delta. This tablet provided the key to the decipherment of Egyptian hieroglyphics.

[21] ultraviolet radiation from the sun (or ionizing radiation such as X-rays), which is largely screened out by the ozone layer now, is carcinogenic, or causes cells to revert back to the way they were billions of years ago, because UV radiation was abundant on the surface of the early Earth (i.e., cancer cells evolved under high UV conditions). UV-screening ozone (O_3) can only be

formed if the atmosphere contains high levels of
oxygen.

[22] natural selection = a survival advantage leading to more
offspring

[23] miso = fermented soybeans used in Japanese
cuisine

[24] endosymbiosis = the absorption of one
species of bacterium into another, so that they
can live togetherand help each other survive

[25] eukaryotic = possessing a distinct nucleus with DNA

[26] plants have tumors, too—a good example is "Crown Gall"
disease in tobacco plants

[27] Cloning creates a group of genetically identical
cells descended from a single common ancestor,
such as a bacterial colony whose members arose
from a single original cell as a result of binary
fission. Source: *Microsoft Bookshelf 2000*

[28] many cancer cells have multiple nuclei, too

[29] mitochondria are tiny bodies inside bacteria
and other cells that are involved in the cell's
energy generating system. Mitochondrial DNA
is totally self-contained and is inherited only
through the mother,unlike DNA in the cell's
nucleus, which is inherited from both parents.

[30] We owe a deep debt of gratitude to *Pelomyxa*
for surviving to the present day to provide us with
much insight into how and when cancer
originated.

[31] Most protists are one-celled and can be seen only with a microscope. Like plants, many species of protists can make their own food by photosynthesis. Like animals, many protists can move around under their own power. The wide variety of protists includes seaweeds, amoebas, and slime molds. All protists are eukaryotes, meaning that their cells contain a nucleus. Most protists have a single nucleus, but some contain multiple nuclei. Many protists are tiny, but giant kelps can grow to 40 m (130 ft) long. [Source: *Microsoft Bookshelf 2000*]

[32] From Zhou, Y. and Lee, A., "Mechanism for the Suppression of the Mammalian Stress Response by Genistein, an Anticancer Phytoestrogen from Soy." JNCI, Vol. 90, No. 5, March 4, 1998.

[33] Venus is much closer to the Sun and has a thicker atmosphere than the Earth. It is so hot (the average surface temperature is 900° Fahrenheit), because of the greenhouse effect created by its 96% CO_2 atmosphere, that lead would melt at its surface. Mars has a much thinner atmosphere (only about 1% of the Earth's) and is much farther away from the Sun. Venus, in fact, resembles the way the early Earth was, while Mars probably resembles how the Earth may look a billion years from now.

BIBLIOGRAPHY
FOR
THE ORIGIN OF CANCER

A

Abrahamson, E. M., and Pezet, A. W. (1951). *BODY, MIND, AND SUGAR.* Avon Books.

Adams, Ruth. (1972, 1976). *THE COMPLETE HOME GUIDE TO ALL THE VITAMINS.* Larchmont Book.

Adams, Ruth. (1976). *EATING IN EDEN.* Rodale Press.

Akasofu, S. I., and Kamide, Y., editors. (1987). *THE SOLAR WIND AND THE EARTH.* Scientific Publications Co. QB529 .S627 (SEL) [SEL = University of California San Diego Science & Engineering Library].

Andreae, M. O., and Schimel, D. S., eds. (1989). *EXCHANGE OF TRACE GASES BETWEEN TERRESTRIAL ECOSYSTEMS AND THE ATMOSPHERE.* John Wiley & Sons. QH344 D131 (BML) [BML = UCSD Biomedical Library].

Arasaki, Seibin, and Arasaki, Teruko. (1983). *VEGETABLES FROM THE SEA.* Japan   Publications, Inc.

Asimov, Isaac. (1987) *BEGINNINGS.* Berkley Press.

Assembly of Life Sciences. (1982). *DIET, NUTRITION, AND CANCER*. National Research Council. National Academy Press.

Atkins, Robert C., and Linde, Shirley. (1977). *DR. ATKINS' SUPER-ENERGY DIET*. Bantam Books.

B

Bahr, Robert. (1976). *THE VIRILITY FACTOR*. G. P. Putnam & Sons.

Bannasch, Peter (ed.) (1988). *CANCER THERAPY*. Springer-Verlag. QZ266 C21473 (BML).

Bartsch, H., Hemminki, K., and O'Neil, I. K. (1987). *METHODS FOR DETECTING DNA DAMAGING AGENTS IN HUMANS - Applications in Cancer Epidemiology and Prevention*. IARC. QW690 M589 (BML).

Bates, Marston. (1964). *MAN IN NATURE*. Prentice-Hall Inc. QH368 B329m (BML).

Becker, Charles E., and Coye, Molly Joel. (1984). *CANCER PREVENTION*. Hemisphere Publishing Corp. (Harper & Row). QZ200 C21575 (BML).

Beeson, Paul B., and McDermott, Walsh. (1975). *TEXTBOOK OF MEDICINE, 14Th EDITION*. W. B. Saunders Co.

Benz, Christopher, and Liu, Edison. (1989). *ONCOGENES*. Kluwer Academic Publishers. QZ202 O574 (BML).

Berger, Stuart. (1989). *FOREVER YOUNG*. William Morrow & Co.

Bierman, June, Toohey, Barbara, and Whitehouse, Fred. (1980). *THE DIABETIC'S TOTAL HEALTH BOOK*. J. P. Tarcher.

Birge, Edward A. (1981, 1988*). BACTERIAL AND BACTERIOPHAGE GENETICS*. Springer- Verlag. QW51 B617B (BML).

Blum, H. F. (1959). *CARCINOGENESIS BY ULTRAVIOLET LIGHT*. Princeton University Press. QZ200 B658c (BML).

Boyden, S. V. (1970). *IMPACT OF CIVILISATION ON THE BIOLOGY OF MAN*. University of Toronto Press.

Boynton, Alton, et al., eds. (1982). *IONS, CELL PROLIFERATION, AND CANCER*. Academic Press. QZ202 S990 (BML).

Bradshaw, Ralph, and Prentis, Steve, eds. (1987). *ONCOGENES AND GROWTH FACTORS*. Elsevier Science Publishing. QZ202 O5793 (BML).

Brewster, Letitia. (1978). *THE CHANGING AMERICAN DIET*. Center for Science in the Public Interest.

Brothers, Milton J. (1976). *DIABETES - THE NEW APPROACH*. Grosset & Dunlap.

Brugge, Curran, Harlow et al. (1991). *ORIGINS OF HUMAN CANCER*. Cold Spring Harbor Press. QZ202 O6952 (BML).

Buick, K. B., Lui, E. X., and Larrick, J. W. (1988). *ONCOGENES*. Springer-Verlag. QZ202 B9480 (BML).

Bullard, Fred M. (1984). *VOLCANOES OF THE EARTH*. University of Texas Press. 551.21 (UCSD Main Library).

Burns, Upton, and Silini, eds. (1984). *RADIATION DNA CARCINOGENESIS AND ALTERATION*. A.S.I. QZ200 N312 (BML).

Butterworth, C.E., Jr. and Hutchinson, Martha L. (1982). *NUTRITIONAL FACTORS IN THE INDUCTION AND MAINTENANCE OF MALIGNANCY*. Bristol-Myers Nutrition Symposia. QZ200 N979 (BML).

C

Caner, Stephen, Olatstein, Eli, and Livingston, Robert. (1982). *PRINCIPLES OF CANCER TREATMENT*. McGraw-Hill. QZ266 P957 (BML).

Carper, Jean. (1988). *THE FOOD PHARMACY*. Bantam Books.

Chaitow, Leon. (1985, 1988). *AMINO ACID IN THERAPY*. Healing Arts Press.

Chamberlain, Joseph, and Hunten, Donald. (1987).
THEORY OF PLANETARY ATMOSPHERES. Academic
Press. QB603 .A85 C48 (SEL).

Cheraskin, E., Ringsdorf, W. M., and Clark, J. W. (1968).
DIET AND DISEASE. Keats Publishing.

Ciegler, Alex, Kadis, Solomon, and Ajl, Samue, eds.
(1971). *MICROBIAL TOXINS*. Academic Press. QW630
M629 V.6 (BML).

Clarke, David H. (1975). *EXERCISE PHYSIOLOGY*.
Prentice-Hall, Inc.

Cleave, T. L. (1974). *THE SACCHARINE DISEASE*. John
Wright & Sons Ltd. QU75 C623s (BML).

Cleton, F. J., and Simons, J., eds. (1980). *GENETIC
ORIGINS OF TUMOR CELLS*. Martinus   Nijhoff
Publishers. QZ200 G328 (BML).

Cold Spring Harbor Laboratory. (1986). *DNA TUMOR
VIRUSES - CONTROL OF GENE EXPRESSION AND
REPLICATION*. Cold Spring Harbor Laboratory. QZ202
C2145 No.4 (BML).

Cold Spring Harbor Laboratory. (1982). *BRANBURY
REPORT 12 - NITROSAMINES & HUMAN CANCER*.
Cold Spring Harbor Laboratory.

Cooper, L., Barber, E., and Mitchell, H. (1968).
NUTRITION IN HEALTH AND DISEASE. Lippincott Co.

Corbett, Thomas. (1977). *CANCER AND CHEMICALS*. Nelson-Hall.

Cousins, Norman. (1979). *ANATOMY OF AN ILLNESS*. W.W. Norton & Co.

Cowdey, E. V. (1968). *ETIOLOGY AND PREVENTION OF CANCER IN MAN*. Appleton- Century-Crafts.

Creasey, William A. (1985). *DIET AND CANCER*. Lea & Febiger.

Crick, Francis. (1981). *LIFE ITSELF*. Simon & Schuster. 577.

D

De Cayeux, André. (1964). *THREE BILLION YEARS OF LIFE*. Stein and Day. QH367 C134t (BML).

De Robertis, E. D. P., and De Robertis, E. M. F., Jr. (1980). *CELL AND MOLECULAR BIOLOGY* - 7th Edition. Saunders College/Holt, Rinehart and Winston. 574.87.

Doetsch, R. N., and Cook, T. M. (1973). *INTRODUCTION TO BACTERIA AND THEIR ECOBIOLOGY*. University Park Press. QW4 D653i (BML).

Doll, Richard & Peto, Richard (1981). *THE CAUSES OF CANCER*. Oxford University Press. QZ202 D665c (BML).

Douglass, William Campbell. (1985). *THE MILK OF HUMAN KINDNESS IS NOT PASTEURIZED*. Copple House Books, Inc.

E

Emanuel, N. M., and Lyaskovskaya, Yu. N. (1967). *THE INHIBITION OF FAT OXIDATION PROCESSES*. Pergamon Press. TP671 E413 (SEL).

Ensminger, M. E. (1976). *BEEF CATTLE SCIENCE*. Interstate Printers & Publishers, Inc.

F

Farmer, Peter B., and Walker, John M., eds. (1985). *THE MOLECULAR BASIS OF CANCER*. John Wiley & Sons. QZ200 M717 (BML).

Feo, Francesco, Pani, Paolo, Columbano, Amedea, and Garcea, Renato, eds. (1987). *CHEMICAL CARCINOGENESIS*. Plenum Press. QZ202 S244 (BML).

Fernholm, Bo, Bremer, Kare, and Jornvall, Hans. (1988). *THE HIERARCHY OF LIFE*. 1988 Excerpta Medica. QH367.5 N744 (BML).

Fischer, David S., and Marsh, John C. (1982). *CANCER THERAPY*. G.K. Hall Medical Publishers. QZ266 P529c (BML).

Fleck, Henrietta. (1976). *INTRODUCTION TO NUTRITION*. Macmillan Publishing Co.

Floch, Martin H. (1981). *NUTRITION AND DIET THERAPY IN GASTROINTESTINAL DISEASE*. Plenum Pub. Corp.

Fox, Martin. (1984). *HEALTHY WATER FOR A LONGER LIFE*. Dunaway Foundation.

Frazier, Claude A. (1974). *COPING WITH FOOD ALLERGY*. N.Y. Times Book Co.

Fredericks, Carlton. (1976). *PSYCHO-NUTRITION*. Putnam Publishing Group

Fryer, Lee. (1986). *THE NEW ORGANIC MANIFESTO*. Earth Foods Associates.

Fryer, Lee. (1982). *THE BIO-GARDENER'S BIBLE*. Chilton Book Co.

Futuyma, Douglas. (1986). *EVOLUTIONARY BIOLOGY*. Sinauer Associates, Inc. Publishers. QH366.2 F996e (BML).

G

Gamer, R. Cohn, and Hradec, Jan, eds. (1988). *BIOCHEMISTRY OF CHEMICAL CARCINOGENESIS*. Plenum Press QZ202 B612 (BML).

Georgakas, Dan. (1980). *THE METHUSELAH FACTORS.* Simon & Schuster.

Gitelman, Hillel (ed.) (1989). *ALUMINUM AND HEALTH.* 1989 Marcel Dekker, Inc. QV65 A471 (BML).

Glassman, Judith. (1983). *THE CANCER SURVIVORS.* Dial Press (Doubleday).

Graham, James. (1992). *CANCER SELECTION.* Aculeus Press. QH366.2 G739 (BML).

Greenwald, Peter, Ershow, Abby, et al. (1985). *CANCER, DIET, AND NUTRITION - A   COMPREHENSIVE SOURCEBOOK.* Marquis Who's Who. QZ202 C2147 (BML).

Greenwald, Howard P. (1992). *WHO SURVIVES CANCER?* U.C. Press. QZ200 G8174W (BML).

Greim, Helmut (ed.), et al. (1982). *BIOCHEMICAL BASIS OF CHEMICAL CARCINOGENESIS.* Raven Press. QZ202 W922 (BML).

Guenzi, W. D. (ed.) (1974). *PESTICIDES IN SOIL & WATER.* Soil Science Society of America, Inc.

Gunstone, F. D. (1967). *AN INTRODUCTION TO THE CHEMISTRY AND BIOCHEMISTRY OF FATTY ACIDS AND THEIR GLYCERIDES.* Chapman & Hall, Ltd. TP671 G976 (SEL).

Gurpide, E., Calandra, R., et al., eds. (1983). *HORMONES AND CANCER*. Alan R. Liss, Inc. QZ200 I616 H812 (BML).

Guyion, Arthur. (1979). *PHYSIOLOGY OF THE HUMAN BODY*. Saunders.

H

Hacker, Miles P., Douple, Evan B., and Krakoff, Irwin H., eds. (1983). *PLATINUM COORDINATION COMPLEXES IN CANCER CHEMOTHERAPY*. Martinus Nijhoff Publishing. QZ267 1616 P716 (BML).

Halliwell and Gutteridge. (1985). *FREE RADICALS IN BIOLOGY AND MEDICINE*. Clarendon Press. QP527 HI9IF (BML).

Hausman, P., and Hurley, J. (1989). *THE HEALING FOODS*. Rodale Press.

Hausman, Patricia. (1983). *FOODS THAT FIGHT CANCER*. Rawson Assoc.

Herbert, R. A., and Codd, G. A., eds. (1986). *MICROBES IN EXTREME ENVIRONMENTS*. Academic Press. QW4 M620 (BML).

Hochachka, Peter W. (1980). *LIVING WITHOUT OXYGEN*. Harvard University Press. QP177 H63 (BML).

Hoffer, Abram, and Walker, Morton. (1978). *ORTHOMOLECULAR NUTRITION*. Keats Publishing, Inc.

Hoffman, Dietrich, and Harris, Curtis S., eds. (1986). *MECHANISMS IN TOBACCO CARCINOGENESIS*. Cold Spring Harbor Laboratory. QZ202 N4864 (BML).

Homma, J. Y., et al. (1984). *BACTERIAL ENDOTOXIN*. Verlag Chemie GmbH. QW630 B129 (BML).

Howland, William S., and Carlon, Graziano C. (1885). *CRITICAL CARE OF THE CANCER PATIENT*. Year Book Medical Publishers. QZ266 C934 (BML).

Hyman, Jane W. (1990). *THE LIGHT BOOK*. Jeremy P. Tarcher, Inc.

I

Ishihara, Takaaki, and Sasaki, Masao S., eds. (1983). *RADIATION-INDUCED CHROMOSOME DAMAGE IN MAN*. Alan R. Liss, Inc. QH462 Al R129 (BML).

Iversen, Olav Hilmar. (1988). *THEORIES OF CARCINOGENESIS*. Hemisphere Publishing Corporation. QZ202 T398 (BML).

J

Johanson, Donald, and Shreeve, James. (1989). *LUCY'S CHILD*. William Morrow and Co., Inc.

Johanson, Donald, and Edey, Maitland. (1981). *LUCY - THE BEGINNINGS OF HUMANKIND*. Simon and Schuster. 569.9.

Jones, Lovell A. (ed.) (1989). *MINORITIES AND CANCER*. Springer-Verlag. QZ200 M666 (BML)

K

Kahn, Patricia, and Graf, Thomas. (1986). *ONCOGENES AND GROWTH CONTROL*. Springer- Verlag. QZ202 0576 (BML).

Kaiser, Hans B. (1981). *NEOPLASMA - COMPARATIVE PATHOLOGY OF GROWTH IN ANIMALS, PLANTS, AND MAN*. Williams & Wilkins. QZ200 N4395 (BML).

Kandler, Otto, and Zillig, Wolfram. (1985). *ARCHAEBACTERIA '85*. Gustav Fischer Verlag. QW4 E535 (BML).

Kavaler, Lucy. (1975). *NOISE - THE NEW MENACE*. John Day Co.

Kira, Alexander. (1976). *THE BATHROOM*. Viking Press.

Kimball, Al, and Oro, J. (1971). *PREBIOTIC AND BIOCHEMICAL EVOLUTION*. North-Holland Publishing Co. QH366 P922 (BML).

Kornberg, Arthur. (1974). *DNA SYNTHESIS*. W.H. Freeman and Co. QP624 K67 (BML).

Kowalski, Robert E. (1989). *THE 8-WEEK CHOLESTEROL CURE*. Harper & Row.

Kozlowski, Lynn T., et al., eds. (1990). *RESEARCH ADVANCES IN ALCOHOL AND DRUG PROBLEMS, VOL. 10*. Plenum Press. WM270 R432 (BML).

Krause, Marie, and Mahan, L. Kathleen. (1984). *FOOD, NUTRITION, AND DIET THERAPY*, 7th Edition. W.B. Saunders Co.

Kropf, William. (1980). *HARMFUL FOOD ADDITIVES*. Ashley Books.

L

Lancaster, H. O. (1990). *EXPECTATIONS OF LIFE*. Springer-Verlag. WA900 L244e (BML).

Landsberg, Helmut E. (1969). *WEATHER AND HEALTH*. Doubleday & Co., Inc.

Laszlo, John. (1987). UNDERSTANDING CANCER. Harper & Row.

Laszlo, John (ed.) (1986). *PHYSICIAN'S GUIDE TO CANCER CARE COMPLICATIONS*. Marcel Dekker, Inc. QZ266 P578 (BML).

Lehmann, Justus F. (ed.) (1990). *THERAPEUTIC HEAT AND COLD*. Williams & Wilkins. WB469 T398 (BML).

Lehrer, Steven. (1979). *ALTERNATIVE TREATMENTS FOR CANCER*. Nelson-Hall. QZ266 L524a (BML).

Lesser, Michael. (1980). *NUTRITION AND VITAMIN THERAPY*. Bantam Books, Inc.

Levenson, Frederick B. (1984). *THE CAUSES AND PREVENTION OF CANCER*. Stein and Day, Inc.

Levitt, Paul M. (1979). *THE CANCER REFERENCE BOOK*. Paddington Press

Levy, Julia, Campbell, Jack J. R., and Blackburn, T. Henry. (1973). *INTRODUCTORY MICROBIOLOGY*. John Wiley & Sons, Inc. QW4 L665I (BML).

Lillyquist, Michael J. (1985). *SUNLIGHT & HEALTH*. Dodd, Mead, & Co.

Lin, E. C. C., Goldstein, Richard, Syyanen, Michael. (1984). *BACTERIA, PLASMIDS, AND PHAGES*. QW5I L735B (BML).

Lister, D., and Rhodes, D., eds. (1976). *MEAT ANIMALS*. Plenum Press. SF95 S989.

Livingston, Virginia. (1972). *CANCER - A NEW BREAKTHROUGH*. Nash Publication. 616.99.

Luria, Salvador E. (1973). *LIFE...THE UNFINISHED EXPERIMENT*. Charles Scribner's Sons QH367 L967 (BML).

Lutes, Frederick, Tarbuck, Edward. (1989). *THE ATMOSPHERE*. Prentice-Hall.

M

Madigan, Michael, et al., eds. (1984). *BROCK BIOLOGY OF MICROORGANISMS, 4th EDITION*. Prentice Hall. QW4 B864B (BML)

Magnus, Knut. (1980). *TRENDS IN CANCER INCIDENCE*. Hemisphere Publishing Corp. QZ200 T792 (BML).

Magrath, Ian T. (ed.) (1990). *THE NON-HODGKIN'S LYMPHOMAS*. Williams & Wilkins. WM525 N809 (BML).

Man, Jean (ed.) (1989). *A REVOLUTION IN BIOTECHNOLOGY*. ICSU Press. 660.6

Margolies, Cynthia P., and McCredie, Kenneth B. (1983). *UNDERSTANDING LEUKEMIA*. Scribner's Sons.

Margulis, Lynn. (1970). *THE ORIGIN OF EUKARYOTIC CELLS*. Yale University Press. QHS81 M33lo (BML).

Marks, Paul (ed.) (1981). *CANCER RESEARCH IN THE PEOPLE'S REPUBLIC OF CHINA AND THE U.S.A.* Grune & Stratton, Inc. QZ206 C755 1980c (BML).

Mayr, Ernst. (2001). *WHAT EVOLUTION IS*. Basic Books.

McBrien, D. C. H., and Slater, T. F., eds. (1981). *FREE RADICALS, LIPID PEROXIDATION AND CANCER*. Academic Press. QZ202 P853 (BML).

McVickar, Malcolm H., and Walker, William M. (1978). *USING COMMERCIAL FERTILIZERS*. Interstate Printers & Publishers, Inc.

Medes, Grace, and Reimann, Stanley (1963). *NORMAL GROWTH & CANCER*. J.B. Lippincott Co. QZ200 M488n (BML).

Milam, James R., and Ketcham, Katherine. (1981). *UNDER THE INFLUENCE*. Bantam Books.

Miller, Sandford A. (ed.) (1980). *NUTRITION & BEHAVIOR*. The Franklin Institute Press. QU145 W926 (BML).

Mindell, Earl. (1985). *VITAMIN BIBLE*. Warner Books.

Minnich, Jerry. (1983). *GARDENING FOR MAXIMUM NUTRITION*. Rodale Press.

Moon, Thomas, and Micozzi, Marc. (1989). *NUTRITION AND CANCER PREVENTION*. Marcel Dekker, Inc. QZ200 N978 (BML).

Moskowitz, Mark A., and Osband, Michael E. (1984). *THE COMPLETE BOOK OF MEDICAL TESTS*. W.W. Norton and Co. 616.075

N

National Research Council. (1980). *RECOMMENDED DIETARY ALLOWANCES, NINTH REVISED EDITION*. Committee on Dietary Allowances, Food & Nutrition Board, National Academy of Sciences.

Nay, R. (1986). *CANCER - AN ENIGMA IN BIOLOGY AND SOCIETY*. Croom Helm & The Charles Press, Publishers. QZ200 N456C (BML).

Nigam, McBrien, & Slater, eds. (1987). *EICOSANOIDS, LIPID PEROXIDATION AND CANCER.* Springer-Verlag. QZ202 E345 (BML).

Nittle, Alan H. (1972). *A NEW BREED OF DOCTOR.* Pyramid House.

Nutrition Review. (1976). *NUTRITION REVIEW'S PRESENT KNOWLEDGE IN NUTRITION, 4th EDITION.* QU145 P933 (BML).

Nutrition Review. (1974, July). *NUTRITION MISINFORMATION AND FOOD FADDISM.*

O

O'Brien, Stephen S. (ed.) (1990). *GENETIC MAPS - Locus Maps of Complex Genomes*. Cold Spring Harbor Laboratory Press. QH445.2 G3282 (BML).

Oberling, Charles. (1952). *THE RIDDLE OF CANCER.* Yale University Press. QZ200 0123R (BML).

Oldham, Robert (ed.) (1987). *PRINCIPLES OF CANCER BIOTHERAPY.* Raven Press. QZ266 P954 (BML).

Oppenheimer, Steven B. (1985). *CANCER - A BIOLOGICAL AND CLINICAL INTRODUCTION.* Jones and Bartlett Publishers. Inc. QZ200 062k (BML).

Ott, John. (1973). *HEALTH AND LIGHT*. The Devin-Adair Co.

P

Parking, Stiller, et al., eds. (1988). *INTERNATIONAL INCIDENCE OF CHILDHOOD CANCER*. IARC. QZ200 I6113 (BML).

Passwater, Richard. (1978). *CANCER AND ITS NUTRITIONAL THERAPIES*. Keats Publishing, Inc.

Passwater, Richard. (1977). *SUPERNUTRITION FOR HEALTHY HEARTS*. Dial Press.

Patterson, H. B. W. (1983). *HYDROGENATION OF FATS AND OILS*. Applied Science Publishers. TP671 737 (SEL).

Pennington, Jean, and Church, Helen Nichols. (1985). *FOOD VALUES OF PORTIONS COMMONLY USED*. Harper & Row.

Perkins and Visek. (1981). *DIETARY FATS AND HEALTH*. American Oil Chemists' Society QU85 D565 (BML).

Perry, Michael C., Yarbro, John W., eds. (1984). *TOXICITY OF CHEMOTHERAPY*. Grune & Stratton, Inc. QZ267 T755 (BML).

Pfeiffer, Carl C. (1978). *ZINC AND OTHER MICRO-NUTRIENTS*. Keats Publishing, Inc.

Pfeiffer, Carl C., and Banks, Jane. (1980). *DR. PFEIFFER'S TOTAL NUTRITION*. Simon and Schuster.

Pique, G. G., et al. (1986). *OMEGA-3, THE FISH OIL FACTORS*. Omega-3 Project, Inc.

Polliak, Aaron (ed.) (1984). *HUMAN LEUKEMIAS - CYTOCHEMICAL AND ULTRASTRUCTURAL TECHNIQUES IN DIAGNOSIS AND RESEARCH*. Martinus Nijhoff . QZ350 H918 (BML).

Ponnamperuma, Cyril (ed.) (1976). *CHEMICAL EVOLUTION OF THE GIANT PLANETS*. Academic Press. QB639 .C46 (SEL).

Powers, Hugh. (1978). *FOOD POWER - NUTRITION & YOUR CHILD'S BEHAVIOR*. Presley.

Prescott, David, and Flexer, Abraham. (1982). *CANCER - THE MISGUIDED CELL*. Charles Scribner's Sons. QZ200 P929c (BML).

Preston, T. R., and Willis, M. B. (1970). *INTENSIVE BEEF PRODUCTION*. Pergamon Press.

Prevention Magazine, eds. (1982). *10 WAYS TO LIVE LONGER*. Rodale Press.

Pritikin, Nathan. (1979). *PRITIKIN PROGRAM FOR DIET & EXERCISE*. Bantam Books.

R

Razin, Aharon, Cedar, Howard, and Riggs, Arthur D. (1984). *DNA METHYLATION - BIOCHEMISTRY AND BIOLOGICAL SIGNIFICANCE*. Springer-Verlag. QP624 D15 (SIO).

Reid, E., Cook, G. M. W., and Morre, D. J., eds. (1982). *CANCER CELL ORGANELLES*. Ellis Horwood Ltd. QZ200 C21406 (BML).

Richard, Dick. (1982). *THE TOPIC OF CANCER*. Pergamon Press. QZ200 RSI4T (BML).

Richard, Victor. (1978). *CANCER, THE WAYWARD CELL*. University of California Press.

Richardson & Stubbs. (1978). *PLANTS, AGRICULTURE, & HUMAN SOCIETY*. W.A. Benjamin, Inc.

Roberts, Leslie. (1984). *CANCER TODAY - ORIGINS, PREVENTION, AND TREATMENT*. Institute of Medicine, National Academy Press. QZ200 R645c (BML).

Rosenbaum, Ernest H., and Rosenbaum, Isadora R. (1980). *A COMPREHENSIVE GUIDE FOR CANCER PATIENTS AND THEIR FAMILIES*. Bull Publishing Co.

Rosenzweig, Mark R., and Leiman, Arnold L. (1982). *PHYSIOLOGICAL PSYCHOLOGY*. D.C. Heath and Co.

Rosner, Louis, and Ross, Shelley. (1987). *MULTIPLE SCLEROSIS*. Prentice-Hall. 616.834.

Ruddon, Raymond. (1981). *CANCER BIOLOGY*. Oxford University Press. QZ200 R914c (BML).

S

Sagan, Dorion, and Margulis, Lynn. (1988). *GARDEN OF MICROBIAL DELIGHTS*. Harcourt, Brace, Jovanovich. 576.

Sagan, Dorion, and Margulis, Lynn. (1986). *MICROCOSMOS*. University of California Press.

Salmon, Sydney (ed.) (1993). *ADJUVANT THERAPY OF CANCER VII*. J. B. Lippincott Co. QZ267 I606 (BML).

Salthe, Stanley N. (1972). *EVOLUTIONARY BIOLOGY*. Holt, Rinehart, and Winston, Inc. QH366.2 S176e (BML).

Sand, L., and Zardi, Luciano, eds. (1983). *THEORIES AND MODELS IN CELLULAR TRANSFORMATION*. Academic Press. QZ202 T396 (BML).

Sattilaro, Anthony. (1982). *RECALLED BY LIFE*. Avon Books.

Sax, N. Irving. (1981). *CANCER CAUSING CHEMICALS*. Van Nostrand Reinhold.

Schleifer, Karl H., and Stackebrandt, Erko. (1985). *EVOLUTION OF PROKARYOTES*. Academic Press. QW51 E936 (BML).

Serrou, B., Schein, P. S., and Imabach, J. L., eds. (1981). *NITROSOUREA IN CANCER TREATMENT*. Elsevier/North-Holland Biomedical Press. QZ267 I616 (BML).

Sheinkin, Schacter & Hutton. (1979). *THE FOOD CONNECTION*. Bobbs-Merril Company, Inc.

Shklovskii, I. S., and Sagan, Carl. (1966). *INTELLIGENT LIFE IN THE UNIVERSE*. Dell Publishing.

Singer, B., and Grunberger, D. (1983). *MOLECULAR BIOLOGY OF MUTAGENS AND CARCINOGENS*. Plenum Press. QZ202 S617m (BML).

Singh, B. N. (1975). *PATHOGENIC AND NON-PATHOGENIC AMOEBAE*. John Wiley & Sons. QX55 A617P (BML).

Slonim, N. Balfour (ed)(1974). *ENVIRONMENTAL PHYSIOLOGY*. C. V. Mosby Co.

Soyka, Fred and Edmonds, Alan. (1977). *THE ION EFFECT*. E. P. Dutton & Co., Inc.

Spinetta, John J., and Deasy-Spinetta, Patricia. (1981). *LIVING WITH CHILDHOOD CANCER*. C.V. Mosby. QZ200 L7858 (BML).

Stafford, H. (1959). *THE EARLY INHABITANTS OF THE AMERICAS*. Vantage Press. E58 S8 (BML).

Stall, Basil A. (ed.) (1979). *MIND & CANCER PROGNOSIS*. QZ200 M663 (BML).

Stanley, Steven M. (1981). *THE NEW EVOLUTIONARY TIMETABLE*. Basic Books, Inc. QH366.2 S789n (BML).

Stewart, Clifford T. (ed.) (1988). *CANCER PREVENTION, DETECTION, CAUSES, TREATMENT*. Hampton Court Press. 616.994.

Stokes, William Lee, Judson, Sheldon, and Picard, M. Dane. (1978). *INTRODUCTION TO GEOLOGY, 2ND EDITION*. Prentice-Hall.

Streffer, Christian (ed.) (1977). *CANCER THERAPY BY HYPERTHERMIA AND RADIATION*. Urban & Schwarzenberg. QZ266 I616 (BML).

Surgeon General. (1979). *SMOKING AND HEALTH - A Report of the Surgeon General*. QV137 S665 (BML).

Sylvester, Edward I. (1986). *TARGET - CANCER*. Charles Scribner & Sons.

T

Taguchi, Tetsuo, and Frei, Emil III, eds. (1990). *CANCER UPDATE*. Excerpta Medica. QZ200 C223 (BML).

Taylor, Joyal. (1988). *THE COMPLETE GUIDE TO MERCURY TOXICITY FROM DENTAL FILLINGS*. Scripps Publishing. 615.9.

Time-Life, eds. (1981). *WHOLESOME DIET*.

Time-Life, eds. (1981). *FIGHTING CANCER.*

Tryfiates, George P., and Prasad, Kedar N. (1987). *NUTRITION, GROWTH, AND CANCER.* Alan R. Liss, Inc. QZ200 I616 N976 (BML).

V

Visser, Margaret. (1986). *MUCH DEPENDS ON DINNER.* Collier Books.

Volk, Wesley, et al. (1986). *ESSENTIALS OF MEDICAL MICROBIOLOGY.* J.B. Lippincott Co. QW4 E783 (BML).

W

Wadsworth, George. (1984). *THE DIET & HEALTH OF ISOLATED POPULATIONS.* CRC Press, Inc. QU146.1 W124D (BML).

Wallace, Bruce. (1966). *CHROMOSOMES, GIANT MOLECULES, AND EVOLUTION.* Norton. QH367 W187c (BML).

Weiner, Michael A. (1981). *THE WAY OF THE SKEPTICAL NUTRITIONIST.* Macmillan Publishing Co.

Weiner, Murray, and Bernstein, I. Leonard. (1989). *ADVERSE REACTIONS TO DRUG FORMULATION AGENTS.* Marcel Dekker, Inc. QV800 W423A (BML).

Weinstein, I. Bernard, and Vogel, Henry S., eds. (1982). *GENES AND PROTEINS IN ONCOGENESIS*. Academic Press. QZ202 O325 (BML).

Whelan, Elizabeth. (1980). *PREVENTING CANCER*. Norton.

Whelan, Elizabeth. (1985). *TOXIC TERROR*. Jameson Books, Inc.

Willcox, Bradley J., Willcox, D. Craig and Suzuki, Makoto. (2002). *THE OKINAWA PROGRAM: HOW THE WORLD'S LONGEST-LIVED PEOPLE ACHIEVE EVERLASTING HEALTH-AND HOW YOU CAN TOO*. Three Rivers Press.

Williams, Chris. (1990). *CANCER BIOLOGY AND MANAGEMENT - AN INTRODUCTION*. John Wiley & Sons. QZ200 W720C (BML).

Williams, Melvin H. (1985). *NUTRITIONAL ASPECTS OF HUMAN PHYSICAL AND ATHLETIC PERFORMANCE*. Charles C. Thomas Publishers. QU145 W725N (BML).

Williams, Sue Rodwell. (1977). *NUTRITION & DIET THERAPY*. C.V. Mosby.

Winick, Myron (ed.) (1977). *NUTRITION AND CANCER*. John Wiley & Sons.

Wurtman, Judith J. (1986). *MANAGING YOUR MIND & MOOD THROUGH FOOD*. Harper & Row.

Z

Zamm, Alfred V. and Gannon, Robert. (1980). *WHY YOUR HOUSE MAY ENDANGER YOUR HEALTH.* Simon & Schuster.

TABLE OF ILLUSTRATIONS

Index

5

The End

of

*The Origin of Cancer
and its Causes and Prevention*